Chased by
the Wolf

This is an outstandingly well-written book that every person with chronic renal disease, end-stage renal disease, or lupus should read. It is also a book that every medical student or future physician should read. *Chased by the Wolf* gives the reader a thorough understanding of the failing kidney and life's choices for care and therapeutic options including transplant-level decisions.

— PAUL E. STANTON JR., MD —

President emeritus of East Tennessee State University
and member of the Tennessee Health Care Hall of Fame

Chased by the Wolf is a captivating story of the almost forty-year marriage of Jill and Fred Sauceman and their battle against what they call "the beast," lupus. It is a personal story, a story of many nights of almost dying from kidney failure only to live on in the hope that one day the beast will be eliminated. If you are fighting your own beast, then read *Chased by the Wolf* and be reminded that no matter how dark it seems, there is always the light of hope.

— Patrick Cronin —

Stage, screen, and television actor and
professor of Theatre and Dance at East Tennessee State University

We dedicate this book
to all the health-care heroes
in Virginia and Tennessee
who made the story possible
and
to those who suffer
from lupus and
chronic kidney disease.

Chased by the Wolf

A LIFE WITH LUPUS AND THE KIDNEY TRANSPLANT THAT SAVED IT

JILL AND FRED SAUCEMAN

Mercer University Press | *Macon, Georgia*
2018

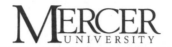

MERCER UNIVERSITY PRESS

Endowed by

TOM WATSON BROWN
and
THE WATSON-BROWN FOUNDATION, INC.

MUP/ P571

© 2018 by Mercer University Press
Published by Mercer University Press
1501 Mercer University Drive
Macon, Georgia 31207
All rights reserved

9 8 7 6 5 4 3 2 1

Books published by Mercer University Press are printed on acid-free paper
that meets the requirements of the American National Standard
for Information Sciences—Permanence of Paper for Printed Library Materials.

Printed and bound in the United States.

ISBN 978-0-88146-671-3 (paperback)
ISBN 978-0-88146-672-0 (ebook)

Cataloging-in-Publication Data is available from the Library of Congress

Book design by Burt&Burt
Text set in Minion Pro and ITC Officina Sans

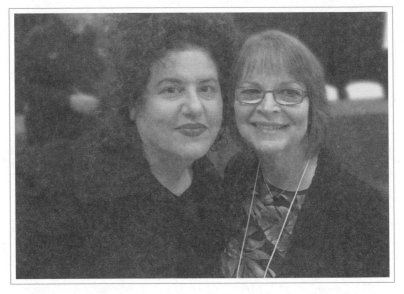

Our friend, author Adriana Trigiani, has followed Jill's story and generously wrote the foreword for this book. Photo by Fred Sauceman.

FOREWORD

— ADRIANA TRIGIANI —

Avid readers of lifestyle and cuisine in the Appalachians can guarantee you the Sauceman family knows their way around a kitchen. Their cornbread, barbecue, biscuits, and gravy are legendary. They present regional cuisine with spectacular flair and a side dish of history.

Now, we learn about Jill and Fred's love story, in *Chased by the Wolf.*

This glorious memoir chronicles Jill's shocking diagnosis of lupus in her youth, and how she copes with an uncertain future. Fred Sauceman, her white knight with a spatula, enters a disco and her life is never the same. The third partner in their vibrant, loving, and complex marriage is Jill's lupus. The co-authors meet the beast head-on, without compromise.

Chased by the Wolf is not only their love story, but an inspirational book about Jill's determination to live a life of purpose despite the diagnosis. They overcome many obstacles together, which is not surprising, but what will delight and amaze the reader is the humor they share, the bond that gives them hope.

The Saucemans may live in the kitchen (and there are those among us who hope they always will), but as you read this very personal story, it will live in your heart. For over 37 years, these lifetime companions, united and strong, have dealt with the worst, but with Jill's fortitude and Fred's love, they keep the beast at bay.

A story of resilience and triumph, put this on the shelf next to your vintage Sauceman collection. You'll turn to it time and again. *Chased by the Wolf* contains the recipe for a happy marriage and the joy that comes from a lifetime commitment.

INTRODUCTION: THE CALL

—— FRED ——

The call came at 1:55 P.M. on Monday, November 10, 2014. The day before, we had helped coordinate the monthly family luncheon at Jonesborough Presbyterian Church in Tennessee's oldest town. Being held in the food-filled month of Thanksgiving, the luncheon drew the year's largest crowd. After the setup, the cooking, and the cleanup, I could tell Jill was exhausted. She was in stage 5 end-stage renal disease, but somehow she got through that luncheon with a smile.

The next day, I was sitting in our sunroom reading the draft of a novel so that I could write a promotional blurb for a friend in West Virginia. Jill was in our den, about 25 feet away. I heard the electronic voice on the answering machine speak the word "Vanderbilt."

We were used to getting calls from the kidney transplant unit at Vanderbilt University Medical Center ever since Jill's first visit there for an evaluation and orientation in August of 2013. But this call seemed different. I could tell she was responding to questions about how she was feeling that day.

I put down the novel and listened intently. The conversation was short, and when it ended, Jill reported it back to me almost verbatim. "Are you running a temperature?" the caller asked. "Do you have transportation to Nashville?" "Can you get here by 10:00 this evening?"

A kidney had become available.

There was an instant rush of elation, of course. But there was no jumping up and down, no prolonged celebration. Throughout this journey, we had both become pretty good at stoicism. The joy of the moment was balanced by the practical needs facing us that day, including a quick trip to Walmart to stock up on necessities, from crackers to extra socks and underwear.

I had almost finalized the text of my afternoon newscasts for public radio station WETS-FM on the campus of East Tennessee State University when that call came. I put the novel aside, made one more quick check of my usual news sources, rushed to the station, recorded the three newscasts that would air later that afternoon, and made arrangements for someone to cover my news for an indefinite period of time, should the promise of a kidney transplant actually come to be. I lined up someone to cover my class, "The Foodways of Appalachia," at a crucial time late in the fall semester.

It was a strange emotional dilemma that November day and evening. We were pulled in all kinds of different directions. We were afraid to rejoice too much—not out of superstition but based on the knowledge that there were still tests ahead and things might not work out. We knew that even a case of the sniffles could derail the whole process, let alone the cross-matching that still needed to take place that night.

In fact, we had gotten a call about an available kidney just nine months before, in February of 2014, and had our bags packed, ready for the four-hour, forty-five-minute drive to Nashville, only to get a call from a transplant coordinator a couple of hours before our planned departure indicating it was a "no go." The surgeon had deemed the kidney unacceptable for transplantation once he had examined it closely after it was removed from the body of a deceased person. The other kidney from that body had been viable, but Jill was second in line. "Emotional rollercoaster" is a cliché, but it aptly describes what transplant candidates go through.

I finished up my work at the radio station the afternoon of November 10, did the Walmart shopping, and returned home, where I learned that a close friend of Jill's family had died. That was one funeral we wouldn't be able to make.

We packed up our new Subaru Forester, which we had just purchased the month before in order to be prepared for driving in snow and ice, and headed west as night was falling. It was a clear but bracing night. As I drove, Jill gathered more information about the transplant procedure via the smartphone and researched the background and education of the transplant surgeon, Dr. Douglas Hale, whom we had not met.

Although we broke no speed limits as we trekked down Interstate 81 and Interstate 40 on the way to Nashville that night, we beat the 10:00 target by an hour. That trip, it would turn out, was a life-changer for both of us—more so than we could ever have imagined. As we'll share in greater detail later in this book, it's a story that still amazes us. We count our blessings every day for the gift of a donated kidney that came our way and the successful transplant that occurred early in the morning of Veterans Day, November 11, 2014. To us, the children of two World War II veterans who managed to survive the fierce fighting in the Pacific Theater of Operations, the Normandy Invasion, and the Battle of the Bulge, that life-saving renal transplant could not have taken place on a more meaningful day.

Without the miraculous gift of a kidney, we could never have walked together to the top of an ancient church in Oxford, England. We could never have kayaked on the Holston River. We could never have attempted to raise Fritz and Sofie, our two lively and endlessly curious miniature schnauzers.

As we documented Jill's experience through the wonder of social media before, during, and after her surgery, we began to think about a book project. With the enthusiastic backing of my longtime publisher, Mercer University Press, that initial idea, conceived on the way home from one of Jill's many follow-up visits to Vanderbilt, took shape. We decided early on that any financial gain we realized through the publication of this book should not be ours. Those funds will be donated to the renal transplant program at Vanderbilt University Medical Center. We remembered that crucial question from the November 10 phone call, "Do you have transportation to Nashville?" And we remembered hearing stories about patients who had to turn down life-saving kidneys because they had no way to travel or no one to accompany them. Any proceeds from the publication of this book will go into a special fund at Vanderbilt to assist transplant patients and their families with transportation and other related expenses.

Our desire to write this book can be reduced to one vital word: hope. If one lupus patient reads these words and realizes that the very serious hardships associated with the disease can be overcome, our work will have been worthwhile. If one person awaiting a kidney transplant finds inspiration and encouragement in our story, making the wait seem a little shorter, the effort will have been valuable to us. Or if a couple in perfect health is struggling to save a marriage, perhaps our story can help keep them together. Strange as it may seem, we think our marriage survived largely because of all the outside pressures against it and because of the people who tried to stop it. We stubbornly made sure it survived to prove those people wrong. Throughout this journey, we have certainly had dark days. We have had days of desperation. We have had days of deep frustration. But I don't recall either of us saying "Why me?" or "Why us?" We never had to look far to find someone in much more dire circumstances than we were experiencing.

Jill and I are people of the mountains. We come from strong stock. Our families, in their own unique ways, have survived and overcome hardships. Their willingness to persevere, to keep fighting, to soldier on is a treasured inheritance. Mountain people don't give up easily. "Can't" is not a part of our mindset. As we will write in a later chapter, we were told that we should not get married. As is the case for many people who grew up in the mountains of East Tennessee and Southwest Virginia, being told we should not or could not do something makes us want to do it all the more. If the marriage survives the process of cowriting this book, we will have been together almost forty years.

It is our hope, too, that the story we share in these pages will encourage more people to consider organ donation.

A SOUTHWEST VIRGINIA CHILDHOOD

—— JILL ——

I am the middle child of three daughters born to Homer and Elsie (Maddux) Derting of Gate City, Virginia. I was born on March 6, 1956, weighing 10 pounds and 13½ ounces. Our home was located in a rural part of Scott County called Brick Yard Gap, between Gate City and Hiltons. My sister Joyce is six years older than I and my sister Janice four years younger. I had a very normal childhood with wonderful parents who always made us feel safe and loved. We didn't have a lot of money for extras, but we had everything we needed and were well fed from all the vegetables grown in my father's garden every year. I grew up in a Christian home, and my parents faithfully served as leaders in our church. I played the piano at church during my high school years, just as my sister Joyce had done before she went to college. When I went to college, my younger sister, Janice, then took over as pianist in that line of succession.

The first memory that I can recall is being in my mother's arms when I was between 1 and 2 at a service at Parker's Chapel Christian Church, named in honor of my paternal grandmother's family. My next memory was when I was 3 years old. I went to Daytona Beach, Florida, with my sister Joyce, my parents, and my maternal aunt Clara Faye and uncle Scott Wood. It was my first experience seeing the ocean.

My paternal grandparents, Martin L. and Nevada (Parker) Derting, lived diagonally across the road from us. Their home was my second home and I was there almost every day. Grandpa Derting's ancestors sailed to America in the 1750s from Amsterdam, but we always understood that the name Derting is German. Grandma Derting's ancestors sailed to America from England. My grandparents raised six boys, and all of them served during World War II. My father served the longest, from 1939 to 1945, and was stationed from 1941 to 1944 in the Pacific Theater of Operations. The other five brothers were in Europe. While he was overseas, my mother worked in the lab at Tennessee Eastman Company in Kingsport, where women filled jobs normally held by the men who were at war. When my father returned home to the States on leave in August of 1944, he and my mother went to the courthouse to get a marriage license. They decided to go ahead and get married while they were there. My father returned to Army bases stateside and was honorably discharged in September of 1945.

Grandpa Derting, who called me "Tadpole," died when I was 5 years old of an aortic aneurysm. He was 77. I don't remember a lot about him, but I do remember him playing the fiddle, rolling his own cigarettes with Prince Albert canned tobacco, and wearing overhauls and a hat. This was my first experience with death, and I couldn't understand why everyone was crying at his funeral. I had been told in Sunday school class that we should rejoice when a loved one enters heaven.

I was very close to Grandma Derting. She taught me to sing alto and to make some of her favorite dishes, including her dried apple stack cake, which she called a "molassee" fruitcake. She would also spend lots of time teaching me how to play Chinese checkers, regular checkers, and card games called Authors and Old Maid, the games of her childhood. Once, when I was visiting her at my uncle Roy's house in Salisbury, North Carolina, where he took care of her during the later years of her life, she told me something that I will always remember.

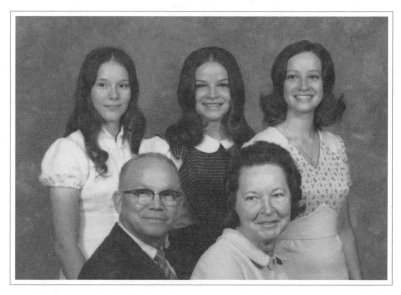

Front row, left to right: Homer and Elsie Derting. Back row, left to right: my sister Janice, me, and my sister Joyce. This picture was taken in 1974, just prior to my hospitalization.

During the fall of 1974, my grandma had to have surgery to remove one-third of her stomach because of a bad ulcer. She knew about the difficulty I was having with my lupus nephritis diagnosis around the same time she entered the hospital. Later that year when I went to see her, she came to me one day while I was getting dressed. She wanted to let me know that I would be okay and that she had prayed to God, telling Him that if He had to take one of us, to please let it be her. She said she had lived her life and mine was just beginning. My grandmother struggled for a while after her surgery, having to adjust to smaller meals more often per day. But she survived the surgery, and I was able to overcome the obstacles that my diagnosis placed in my way. So we both agreed that God wasn't through with either of us at that point.

In December of 1975, she made a final trip back to her Southwest Virginia home. I knew when she came in the door that she was really sick. She spent the Christmas and New Year's holidays with my family, although she was not able to get out of bed. In January, she was admitted to Holston Valley Community Hospital in Kingsport, where she passed away a month later of liver cancer at the age of 85.

My maternal grandparents, Flanders H. and Lona (McNutt) Maddux, were of Scots-Irish heritage. They raised eight children, with my mother being fifth in line. Aunt Sue was the last born and was only 6 months old when my grandmother Maddux died at 42. My mother was 12 at the time and tells me that the doctor said my grandmother died of strep throat. Because of her weakened immune system while taking care of a newborn and several other small children, her throat swelled shut, causing her death. Days earlier, my grandmother's complaint of not being able to swallow fell on the deaf ears of two different doctors. When it appeared that she was dying, the family requested another home visit from her doctor. By the time the doctor could make a house call, there was nothing he could do. I have always wondered if the doctor made a proper diagnosis. But with a home visit, it was probably his best guess for 1934.

All through the years, the close-knit Maddux siblings, along with their spouses and children, would gather at my grandfather Maddux's home for every holiday and for his birthday. We always had fun attending holiday picnics in the apple orchard during the spring and summer months—Memorial Day, the Fourth of July, and Labor Day.

My aunt Uva Maddux was one of 200 people injured in the October 4, 1960, explosion at Tennessee Eastman Company in Kingsport. It was one of the worst days in East Tennessee history. Sixteen people died. My aunt, who never married, was permanently disabled from the accident. She lived with and took care of my grandfather until he died of congestive heart failure in 1969 at age 81. To this day, the F. H. Maddux descendants still gather for birthdays and for Fourth of July and Labor Day picnics.

My mother, 94 at the time of this writing, is the only survivor from her generation.

When I was 5, Aunt Uva provided funds for me to attend kindergarten at First Baptist Church in Gate City, at a time when the public schools in Scott County weren't offering kindergarten instruction. I learned my ABCs, learned to write my name, learned arts and crafts, played games, and sang lots of songs. When our kindergarten graduation came around at the end of the school year, I was chosen to sing "I'm a Little Teapot" and recite the Preamble to the Constitution.

I entered first grade at Hiltons Elementary School during the fall of 1962. Mrs. Ruby Stewart was my teacher. My aunt Claudia Derting taught piano lessons at the elementary school, so I began taking piano that year and continued those lessons through tenth grade. Hiltons Elementary included first through eighth grades, and then students transferred to Gate City High School. At Hiltons I did well in my studies but was most proud of the fact that I had perfect attendance for six of those eight years. Except for normal childhood communicable illnesses in first grade and strep throat in third, I didn't miss a day of school until my junior year in high school. I loved going to school and looked forward every summer to beginning the next school year.

My second-grade teacher, Mrs. Clara Sloan, entered several students in a county-wide talent show. I performed a recitation called "Questions" while dressed in character as a tomboy and won first place for my age category. As a reward, I got to appear on WJHL-TV in Johnson City, as part of "The Virgil Q. Wacks Show." All the top talent-show winners performed their acts on TV that day. My sister Joyce also won first place in her category and got to perform her winning recitation with me.

During my years at Hiltons Elementary, I participated in many extracurricular activities, including 4-H, Girl Scouts, and Glee Club. All those organizations helped me to develop into the person I am today. I will be forever grateful to the teachers, sponsors, and leaders who voluntarily gave their time so that students had the opportunity to learn important life skills from each of those programs. The Hiltons Elementary Glee Club, under the direction of our teachers Paul and Dorothy Argoe, appeared on television when I was in fifth grade, and we also performed every year for the community at Christmas and in the spring. My grandmother Derting's instructions for singing alto came in handy since that is what I was assigned to sing in Glee Club.

Our elementary school had the best softball program in the county. Each grade from fifth through eighth had its own team, and we traveled to or hosted other schools in the county for games. My position on our team was second base, but I was also the relief pitcher. During the summer months, all the children in my neighborhood would get together and play softball in our back yard in order to keep in practice.

During my high school years, I continued to participate in many extracurricular activities and academic organizations. Softball was replaced with football as my sport to support. I attended all the games as an enthusiastic fan. Our football program at Gate City was tops in the county, region, and state, going several years undefeated and winning multiple Virginia State AA championships.

I was active in our high school chorus, making All-Regional Chorus my sophomore, junior, and senior years and All-State Chorus my senior year. I had switched from alto to second soprano and continued to sing that part all through high school and through college at East Tennessee State University, where I was a member of the ETSU Choir.

I was an honor student who was good at most subjects, but I liked math and science the best, particularly math. My high school English composition teacher, Hazel Culbertson, once told me that I wrote like a mathematician, just like I was solving a problem. At the end of my senior year, I was chosen to receive the math award, following in my sister Joyce's footsteps. Courses that I selected to prepare me for the nursing curriculum in college included Algebra I and II, Algebra III and Trigonometry, Geometry, Biology, and Chemistry. I even took two years of Latin to help me with the medical terms which are rooted in that language. In my adult years, I have developed a love of history, realizing it is much more than memorizing facts and dates.

I graduated fourth in my high school class with big plans for the future. I always knew I would go on to college. Neither of my parents attended college, but they were academically capable of doing so. They never pushed college on my sisters and me, but somehow I knew it was expected of us, and it was something that I wanted for myself. All three of the daughters earned college degrees.

My mother was a homemaker during the years when my sisters and I were growing up. She saw to our every need, cooked wonderful meals, was a great seamstress, and was skilled in arts and crafts. She helped our elementary school classes as a homeroom mother, served as a Brownie Girl Scout leader, and supported the local Girl Scout camp.

Mama never learned to drive, which was not unusual for rural women of her generation. My father always graciously got us to wherever we needed to be. As Fred and I complete this book, my mother continues to thrive. She still lives by herself and is in fairly good health. Her biggest limitation is macular degeneration, which is causing her slowly to lose her eyesight.

Daddy loved people. He never met a stranger and would strike up a conversation anywhere, including with people in the doctor's waiting room when I would go for my appointments. He loved hauling us and neighbor children around when we went to Girl Scout meetings or band practices. Daddy just loved to be on the go and do for others. I inherited my singing ability from his side of the family. Not only was he the song leader at church, but he also sang bass with his mother and two brothers, as the Derting Quartet. When he served our country during World War II, his rank was technical sergeant. Part of his job was to service airplanes flying between Australia/New Guinea and Japan and surrounding islands. Naturally, he was always a fix-it person, and I learned that particular skill by following him around all the time while he was working on a project. My mother-in-law always told the story about coming to our home and finding Fred in the kitchen cooking and me on the bathroom floor, fixing the commode.

My father would pass away too soon at the age of 72. His death in 1992 was attributed to cardiac arrhythmia. It was a shock to the whole family, especially since he seemed to be the healthiest of all his brothers. Four of his five brothers died of heart disease.

I don't think there was ever a day during my childhood that I felt lonely or lacked something to do. I jumped at the chance to go somewhere or do something with family and friends. But the lupus diagnosis would change all that.

My loving husband has always been an inspiration to me, encouraging me to try new things and go beyond my limits, knowing that I was (and am) capable of doing such things without any fear. His many years of love and support have been the driving force behind my zest for life and not giving in to my illness. Whether I was feeling sick, in pain, or lying in a hospital bed seriously ill, he was always there by my side. Many lupus patients do not have successful relationships or marriages. Spouses and significant others often tire of their loved one feeling bad all the time and choose to leave. But we chose to believe that every bad moment would eventually end and our lives would be back to normal again. Normal...I really don't think I knew what it was like to feel normal until after my kidney transplant. I thought I always had plenty of energy to do the things I wanted to do. Instead, I learned to live in the moment, finding the energy to do things and then crashing until I had rested enough to go again. This had become the normal life for me until November 2014. I suppose Fred had adjusted to my life being this way, too. There have been moments of frustration for both Fred and me, but we are committed to our marriage and take the vow "in sickness and in health" seriously. I couldn't have asked for a better partner.

In the forty-three years I have lived with lupus and chronic kidney disease, I never lost my faith in God—never through the lupus nephritis diagnosis; never through the many times I was hospitalized or neared death's door; and never through my kidneys failing or desperately searching for a kidney donor. God was always there to pull me through, and I'm definitely a believer in prayer and in miracles. I've never once stopped to ask, "Why me, Lord?" I felt that I was given this illness because God knew that I had faith in Him to see me through it. This faith is a defining part of my life.

2

THE MEETING

—— FRED ——

Life can turn on the simplest of decisions. My choice of where to go after a football game would change the trajectory of my life forever. It was the fall of 1978. The previous spring, I had graduated from East Tennessee State University with a Bachelor of Arts degree in English and History. I entered graduate school that fall to pursue a Master of Arts degree in English.

ETSU, however, wasn't my first choice after high school. In the fall of 1974, I had entered the University of Tennessee in Knoxville. Scholarship offers came in from other schools, but it was a foregone conclusion that I would go to UT. I had always followed the school's athletic program, and, although I graduated from Greeneville High School in Greeneville, Tennessee, whose students overwhelmingly ordered class rings with green stones, mine was orange. One of my best friends, Ben Britton, whom I had known since toddlerhood through Asbury United Methodist Church, became my roommate. (Ben would die of ALS, Lou Gehrig's Disease, on November 30, 2015.) Both of Ben's parents were living—active and vibrant—when we entered UT that fall. I didn't have that luxury.

On a gorgeous fall afternoon in October of 1971, while I was on the tennis court, my father, for whom I am named, was stricken while mowing the yard. He had a violent seizure, and how he managed to get through it without being cut to pieces on our sloping yard by his riding lawn mower is still hard for me to fathom. My mother managed to get him to the hospital, and I still remember her telling me about frantically trying to get him help while a clerk at the hospital spent precious minutes questioning her about insurance. My father was transferred by ambulance to Memorial Hospital in Johnson City and underwent a spinal tap that evening. The spinal fluid contained no blood, and the neurologist released him a couple of days later without a diagnosis.

Meanwhile, my father began to suffer from increasingly severe headaches. My mother convinced our family doctor in Greeneville to refer him to Vanderbilt University Medical Center, where, in January of 1972, he was diagnosed with a brain tumor. Surgery was performed to remove a golf-ball-sized tumor over his ear. It was malignant, the doctor informed us. But for some reason, we did not tell my father. I think he suspected, especially after he was subjected to cobalt treatments back in Greeneville. But we never used the "C" word in front of him. The hope we held out for him, I realize now, was false. We would grasp onto any kind of encouragement we could. I still remember the night when my father, who had made radios, phonographs, and televisions for the Magnavox Company, rewired my stereo, about three months after his brain surgery. We celebrated that moment.

But those instances of hope were rare, and by midsummer of 1972, his headaches had returned. I will never forget the tearful night when my mother finally had to tell him that his brain had been invaded by cancer. It was probably the only time in my life when I had seen him cry. He demanded to see one of his sisters, Selma Overbay, although he hadn't been in close contact with her for years. We called her at 3:00 that morning, and she came.

My father's decline from that point on was relentless. By the fall of 1972, almost exactly a year after the first seizures, he had begun to experience falls. My mother, who had worked full-time for a dress factory before I was born and part-time for the United Fund and in the tobacco market in Greeneville after I started elementary school, was without steady employment. Her full-time job was caring for my father. But she couldn't do it alone and

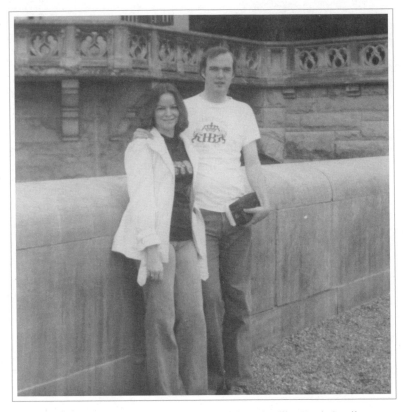

This picture was taken at Biltmore Estate in Asheville, North Carolina, shortly after we met.

somehow managed to scrape together the money to hire a sitter, a man named "Boat" Douthat, who was experienced in lifting helpless patients. The three of us watched as my father, once an active man of 200 pounds, lost half his body weight and went blind.

The year before, at the suggestion of my mother, I had applied for a job at one of the local radio stations in Greeneville, WGRV, and was hired, even though, at age 15, I couldn't drive a car and had to be taken to work by my mother. After disc-jockeying rock-and-roll shows on Saturday nights and Sunday nights, I would call my mother at about 12:30 in the morning to tell her I was ready for a ride home. She always arrived without complaint, despite the terrible burden she was dealing with at home.

By the summer of 1972, I had my driver's license and was able to relieve my mother of at least that one responsibility. On Sunday night, January 7, 1973, I had worked my usual shift and had driven home in a snowstorm. The next morning, we noticed that my father's legs were slowly turning black. By that afternoon, he was gone. The driveway was so icy on that January 8 that the hearse couldn't get close to the house. My father's body had to be taken across our snowy yard.

I grew up knowing all four of my grandparents and both my parents, but by the time I was sixteen years old, my mother, Wanda Sauceman, was the only one of the six still alive. Those encounters with death at an early age have largely defined my life. And they help explain my mother's reactions when she began to learn some of the details of Jill's life.

Being widowed at age 49 was something my mother never got over. While I loved the University of Tennessee and succeeded there, my mother was falling apart. I would call her from my dormitory once a week, and those calls always resulted in her tears. I came home every weekend. I had no brothers or sisters to call on for help.

Academic life at the University of Tennessee had opened up new worlds for me. I took courses in its famous Department of Anthropology. I studied under one of the grand old men of the Department of Geology, Dr. James G. Walls. Best of all, I found a mentor, Dr. F. DeWolfe Miller, professor of English. Although I had graduated as valedictorian of my high school class, I wasn't sure college was for me. I found myself in Dr. Miller's Honors English Composition class that fall quarter of 1974, full of self-doubt. We wrote our first essay in class on a Friday, and I worried all weekend about how I had done. When Dr. Miller handed my paper back to me the following Monday, he had written in the margin, "Sauce, man. A+." That brief comment gave me the confidence to stay in school and one day to become a writer.

I would sit in Dr. Miller's office on the UT campus for hours, listening to his stories about writers he knew and about his days as an FBI agent. I would go on to take two other courses with him, one in American humor.

I was torn between the joys of the classroom at UT and the need to attend to my grieving mother. In the fall of 1975, I made the decision to leave the University of Tennessee, take my old job back at radio station WSMG in Greeneville, and transfer to East Tennessee State University in Johnson City that next spring. I would ultimately find a meaningful place on the ETSU campus, where I have remained, as student, administrator, and professor, ever since. For the rest of my undergraduate years, I lived with my mother and commuted back and forth to Johnson City.

I never regretted my decision to transfer. My professors at ETSU were superb, guiding me through a liberal arts education that I deeply value to this day. And for the purposes of this story, it's important to point out that had I not continued my education at ETSU, there is a very high likelihood that I would never have met Jill Marie Derting.

By the summer of 1978, I had been in radio about seven years and felt it was time to try television. I landed a job at WKPT-TV in Kingsport, Tennessee, where I did field reporting and some anchor work while taking graduate-level courses in English and teaching two classes in English composition as a graduate assistant. Part of my responsibilities at WKPT involved recording a 30-second newsbreak on Saturday evenings, sponsored by Tri-City Bank. During "Love Boat" and "Fantasy Island," I'd appear for half a minute to provide a summary of Tennessee and Virginia headlines.

But on Saturday night, September 30, 1978, I had arranged for someone else to cover those newsbreaks so I could attend the East Tennessee State University versus Western Kentucky University football game in Johnson City with my longtime friend Joe Seaton. Joe and I had been friends since first grade days at East View Elementary School. He, too, is an only child. Joe and I stayed until the end of the game, which ETSU lost by a score of 27–21.

The direction of my entire life would change that night. The simple decision about where two college guys should go after a ball game altered the course of my very existence.

With the legal drinking age at 18, there were lots of choices for evening entertainment in Johnson City back then—among them a cavernous beer hall called the Tu La Fe near the ETSU campus, the Crow's Nest, and the Ambassador Lounge. It was the disco era, when dance music dominated as the nation tried to forget the divisiveness of the Vietnam War and the disappointment and disillusionment of the Watergate scandal. "I love the night life, I got to boogie, on the disco 'round, oh yeah," sang Alicia Bridges in one of 1978's most popular and carefree dance numbers.

Johnson City even had a discotheque in its shopping mall. It was called Super Wheels, and it was elbow-to-elbow and hip-to-hip on Friday and Saturday nights. Of all the establishments we had to choose from in town, Super Wheels was the place Joe and I visited after that home football game.

When people ask Jill and me how we met and I say, "She tripped over me in a bar," it's really no exaggeration. That's literally what happened. I was kneeling on the floor at a table talking to a classmate from high school, Robin Webb, when Jill returned to the table and slightly stumbled over my size-12 shoe stretched out in the middle of the floor. Jill had a headache that night and didn't want to go out, but Robin convinced her to get out of the dorm room and go. Again, life turns on the most minor of decisions.

Robin and Joe went up to dance, leaving Jill and me at the table by ourselves. A few moments of silence passed before Jill introduced herself. I took it as a good sign that she spoke first. She had recognized me from my appearances on the news at WKPT-TV. Soon we made our way to the dance floor, and conversation got easier. Seeing that we were hitting it off, Joe, who had ridden to the disco with me, decided to hitch a ride with Robin back to the campus, leaving Jill with no transportation. His plan worked. Jill had no choice but to ride back to campus with me. We sat in the car that night and talked until 4:00 in the morning.

Keep in mind that I was still living at home at that time, so I arrived back in Greeneville at 5:00 in the morning. "Any girl who would stay out until 4:00 in the morning isn't worth much," my mother declared over a late breakfast of salt-risen bread and tea the next day.

Jill and I had our first official date at Augustino's, a magnificent Italian restaurant run by a Lebanese family in my hometown. The night we first met, we discovered that we both liked Italian food. Augustino's was the best around. I can still remember what I had on that first date: a plate of house-made Italian sausage, scaloppini of beef Marsala, and Arabic rice.

Since UT had been a suitcase college for me, I was ready to immerse myself in the social life of a college campus that fall. As my relationship with Jill deepened, my desire to spend more time in Johnson City intensified. I found a small apartment just outside Kingsport, a ten-minute drive to WKPT and a twenty-minute drive to the ETSU campus. In short, I began doing what most 22-year-olds do: developing a serious relationship and establishing some independence. When I came back home to Greeneville one night and began collecting items to furnish that apartment, my mother unraveled. It was one of the first and one of the worst confrontations we had ever had.

Meanwhile, Jill and I were spending more and more time together. Many of our dates would begin and end in Carter Hall, the most charming of all the women's residence halls at ETSU. It is one of two original buildings still standing on campus, and it has remained true to its initial purpose, to house women students. The building opened in the fall of 1911, as the first twenty-nine students enrolled at what was then East Tennessee State Normal School. The brick structure at the center of the campus has a parlor with a grand piano. Every night, that parlor would be filled with coeds and their dates.

Behind the front desk, in a small apartment, lived Carter Hall's dorm mother, Marguerite Keefauver, a stately, white-haired lady with a perpetual smile who stood in quiet judgment to approve or disapprove every boyfriend who dated a Carter Hall inhabitant. She was one of the defining personalities of the campus, and she loved "her girls." When Mrs. K. found out I was on TV, she would allow Jill to come back to her private apartment and watch my newscasts. When Jill and I married, we had no surviving grandparents. Mrs. K. became the honorary grandmother in our wedding. She would have remained in her job as the last dorm mother on campus for many years longer, but state-mandated retirement forced her out of that job when she attained the age of 70.

About a month after I met Jill, we were talking in my car outside Taylor Hall, a men's residence on the ETSU campus (that has since been demolished), when I sensed that it was time to say something I had been thinking ever since the night we met. I told her that I loved her.

Then there were tense seconds of silence. And she said, "Oh, no."

That unanticipated reply was followed by more silence. And then she said, "There's something about me I think you need to know." My mind quickly began to construct possible scenarios of a jaded past. But through her need to explain her shocking response, I began to learn the details of what had been, up to that point, a secret story she had kept hidden inside her. She had withheld that story from me in hopes that our relationship would not suddenly end, as others had for her.

3

THE DIAGNOSIS

—— JILL ——

Ever since working as a candy striper at Holston Valley Community Hospital in Kingsport, Tennessee, I had wanted to be a nurse. I don't believe candy stripers exist anymore. At least the striped uniforms don't. They're just called volunteers now. Among other duties, I would fill patients' water pitchers, deliver specimens from surgery to the laboratory, and transport patients to and from physical therapy. I even worked as a waitress in the hospital's grill. Being in the hospital setting confirmed my decision to become a nurse. East Tennessee State University was my first choice for nursing school. Its programs had and continue to have an impressive reputation. And despite the fact that residents of Scott County, Virginia, where I lived, had to pay out-of-state tuition, ETSU was still an educational bargain. Many people in Southwest Virginia viewed ETSU as the regional university for that part of the state then, and they still feel that way.

I was required to undergo a physical examination before enrolling at ETSU. I scheduled that examination for August 20, 1974. I had graduated from Gate City High School in Gate City, Virginia, at the end of May. After graduation, I went camping in Myrtle Beach, South Carolina, with my Girl Scout leaders and the other senior members of the troop. I remember counting sixty-two mosquito bites on my arms and legs alone and ended up sleeping in our leader's car for most of that trip. I found it extremely strange that no one else in our group had gotten attacked by so many mosquitoes.

When I got home, I felt really tired and sluggish. One day in June, I went to the bathroom and the urine was the color of dark tea. I would sleep that summer until 10:00, get up, move to the couch, and watch television. I didn't feel like doing anything else.

I did agree to take my disabled aunt to visit my cousin's newborn baby in Christiansburg, Virginia. My aunt, Uva Maddux, was the one who had been so badly injured in the Tennessee Eastman explosion in 1960. She was working as a secretary there when a metal pipe took about four inches of bone out of one leg and lodged in the other. She used her dress as a tourniquet to stop the bleeding and had to crawl off the floor to the top of a desk to escape leaking acid on the floor. Doctors were able to save her leg, and when she got home, nurses came to visit. I saw them in action when I was 4 years old, and I decided that becoming a nurse should be my career path.

At any rate, Aunt Uva asked me to take her to Christiansburg that summer of 1974. I didn't feel like making the trip, but she had been so good to me that I felt I couldn't turn her down. She could drive locally with the help of some special equipment that had been added to her car, but an overnight trip was impossible for her. I drove her to Christiansburg, feeling bad the entire time. I spent the night in the bathroom nauseated. The next morning, we came home, and I had to drive with the worst headache I've ever had in my life. I kept thinking that I couldn't make it home quick enough. When we got close to Bristol, she decided that she wanted to go shopping at King's Department Store and I took her, not letting on that I had such a terrific headache. When we got home, I crashed.

I went back to my routine of sleeping until 10:00. My parents would call me lazy. I didn't feel like preparing my things for college. And I continued to ignore the tea-colored urine. For that college physical at a health clinic in Nickelsville, Virginia, the first thing I did was to provide a urine specimen, and it looked just like dark tea. I saw the look on the lab technician's face, which confirmed that something was seriously wrong. When I saw our family physician, Dr. Jerry Miller, he told me I might have Bright's Disease

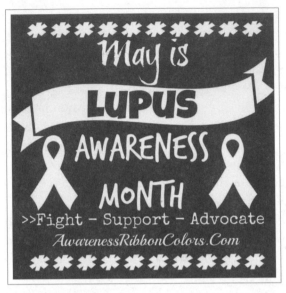

Still, so many people in America are unfamiliar with lupus.
We can change that. Source: Lupus Foundation of America.

and that I should enter the hospital immediately. He told me to go
home, get my things together, and report to Holston Valley Community Hospital in Kingsport for admission. Suddenly my college
future was in doubt.

A cystoscopy was performed, which involved exploration of
the bladder and ureters to see if the bleeding was limited to one
kidney or if it was coming from both. The procedure indicated that
both kidneys were indeed involved. Dr. Miller consulted with an
internal medicine physician in Kingsport to figure out what could
be done to decrease the inflammation to stop my kidneys from
bleeding so severely while they determined a diagnosis. Blood
work also showed that I was severely anemic.

I was placed on 80 milligrams of prednisone, and within a
week, even though blood was still in the urine, it was no longer
dark in color. Blood was drawn for testing over a period of several

days. One day Dr. Miller came into my hospital room and said, "We've determined it's not Bright's Disease, and I wish it were."

I had been in the hospital two weeks, still without a definitive diagnosis. My older sister, Joyce, was getting married on August 31, and I begged Dr. Miller to let me participate in the wedding as a bridesmaid. I had purchased my dress in early summer. He gave me a day pass, but after two weeks of being in a hospital bed, I was so weak I couldn't make it down the aisle and had to sit on the front pew of Weber City Baptist Church.

While I was in the hospital, Dr. Miller received a medical journal. In it, there was an article about lupus, an autoimmune disease. He suspected that I might have it and told me there was only one place in the country then that could perform the proper blood test for a lupus diagnosis. He packed up blood samples and sent them there as I waited in the hospital for two more weeks. The results came back positive for lupus nephritis. My doctors got together and determined that prednisone was what I needed to be taking, because there was not a specific treatment for lupus at that time. Most treatments were experimental.

When I was discharged from the hospital in September, it was clear that entering ETSU that fall quarter would be impossible. Now my life was overtaken by a disease I had never even heard of until my family doctor's accurate diagnosis that summer.

After word of my condition got around Scott County, I began getting telephone calls of support. One was from Frances Ann Culbertson, my high school World Geography teacher. She told me that she, too, had lupus, having been diagnosed in the 1940s. Doctors had tried various experimental drugs with her, including gold treatments. The type of lupus she had must have affected her skin. She wore a wig all the time, and the skin on her face had the appearance of crinkled leather. She told me that if she walked even the short distance from the high school to the Campus Drive-In restaurant nearby, she became wobbly and unstable on her feet because of balance problems. Mrs. Culbertson was the first person

I ever knew to have lupus, but I had been totally unaware of it when I was in her high school class.

THREE KEY INDICATORS OF KIDNEY FUNCTION

Urea nitrogen is a waste product that results from the breakdown of protein in the body. **Blood urea nitrogen (BUN)** is measured through a blood test. BUN readings are based on milligrams of urea nitrogen per 100 milliliters of blood. A normal BUN runs between 7 and 20. As kidney function decreases, BUN increases.

Creatinine is a chemical waste product that is generated from muscle metabolism. In normal kidneys, most of it is filtered out and eliminated through the urine. Creatinine is measured in milligrams per deciliter of urine. Depending on a person's age, sex, and muscle mass, a normal creatinine range could be around 0.84 to 1.21.

GFR stands for **glomerular filtration rate**. It measures how well the kidneys are filtering the blood. The National Kidney Foundation says it is the best test to measure kidney function to determine a person's stage of kidney disease. Measured in milliliters per minute, it indicates how much liquid and waste are passing from the blood through the glomeruli—the tiny filters in the kidney—and out into the urine during each minute.

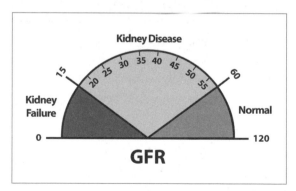

(*Courtesy of the National Institute of Diabetes and Digestive and Kidney Diseases.*)

I spent the late summer and early fall at home, seeing Dr. Miller sometimes as often as twice a week for checkups and blood work. I was still experiencing severe anemia from the months of blood loss from my kidneys. During one appointment in October, Dr. Miller had my parents come into the exam room. He told them that even though the bleeding had been controlled considerably, my creatinine and blood urea nitrogen (BUN) readings were worsening. He felt that I needed to go to a place that specialized in kidney transplants and where I could be placed on the proper medication. In addition, I was having serious side effects from the prednisone, including high blood pressure, weight gain, and elevated blood sugar.

Dr. Miller recommended Vanderbilt University, Duke University, and the Medical College of Virginia. Because I lived in Virginia and because Dr. Miller had graduated from MCV and had connections there, I decided to go to Richmond. That was in late October. My parents did not own a car capable of making the trip, so my uncle and aunt, Earl and Maxie Derting, drove my parents and me to Richmond in their station wagon.

When they found out I was going to have to go to Richmond, neighbors and churches donated money to us to help with the expenses. We got help from my home church, Weber City Christian Church, and from Nottingham United Methodist Church, Hiltons United Methodist, Mount Vernon United Methodist, and the Hiltons Church of God. The Community Chest and Virginia Vocational Rehabilitation Services pitched in to help us as well. Our neighbor, the late Pam Pippin, a year older than I, knocked on neighbors' doors to ask for donations.

When I arrived in Richmond and checked in, I discovered that there was a special outpatient clinic, similar to a hotel, where we could stay. The next day I had an appointment with Dr. Ron Irby, who was a specialist in connective tissue diseases; rheumatologist is the term commonly used today. After reviewing all of the information Dr. Miller had sent him, he pretty much confirmed that it was probably lupus. He coordinated my care there with a nephrologist, a gastroenterologist, and a pulmonologist in order to determine what type of lupus I had and the extent of the kidney damage.

I went through days and days of x-rays, scans, and blood tests, and the doctors determined that a kidney biopsy was in order. Keep in mind that this was 1974 technology. An x-ray was taken to determine the location of the kidneys. After looking at the x-ray, the medical personnel pinpointed what they hoped was the spot by counting so many fingers over from the vertebrae and ribs. It was a risky procedure. There was a chance of hitting an artery, damaging a kidney, and losing the organ. But it was the only way the doctors could determine how badly the lupus had damaged my kidneys and then figure out the proper treatment.

My mother was with me, and she tried to talk me out of having the procedure. I, however, agreed with the doctors that the biopsy should be performed. Dr. David Goldman was the head nephrologist, and he had four other nephrologists working with him on my case. At that point, I left the clinic and entered the hospital as an inpatient for the needle biopsy. "While you were in surgery for the kidney biopsy, I spent my time in the chapel upstairs, praying to God to help the doctors find a medication to make you better," my mother recalls.

After the biopsy, I went back to the clinic, where the doctors made a visit to my room. The final diagnosis was systemic lupus erythematosus, SLE, with diffuse proliferative glomerulonephritis. A mouthful for sure. Seven words, twenty-six syllables—all pretty much foreign to me up to that point. But those words would define and shape most of the rest of my life. To put it simply, the ability of my kidneys to filter my blood had been seriously compromised. With the extent of the lupus damage that had been done, the doctors said they would not be surprised if I would be on dialysis or on a renal transplant list within ten to fifteen years. As it would turn out, I made it almost forty.

The doctors in Richmond decided to prescribe a drug called Imuran, which had only been on the market in America for two years. On a daily dosage of 100 milligrams, I headed back to my parents' house in Scott County, Virginia.

"On the way back home, during the night, you went to the bathroom and said there was blood in your urine," my mother remembers. "We called MCV the next morning, and they said when we got home for you to lay on your back with ice packs for twenty-four to forty-eight hours to give the area time to heal."

In addition to checkups every three to four months back at MCV in Richmond, I saw Dr. Miller weekly for blood tests to determine how well my system was tolerating this new drug. By March of 1975, I had stopped taking prednisone and was finally able to begin my freshman year at East Tennessee State University, although my delay in enrolling had caused me to lose my nursing scholarships. Fortunately, I was able to get financial help from Virginia Vocational Rehabilitation as well as a Basic Educational Opportunity Grant (BEOG), later known as the Pell Grant.

I was elated to be able to begin college. However, the once out-going teenager involved in countless extracurricular activities in high school became a hermit at the beginning of my first quarter at ETSU. From having been on such a large dosage of prednisone, I had developed a severe case of acne. My cheeks were oozing constantly, and I was very self-conscious and embarrassed to be seen at college looking like that. And I still had the "moon face" that prednisone causes. So except for going to class and going to eat, I stayed holed up in my room. I just wanted to lie on my bed and study. As the acne improved, though, I began to take a more active part in campus life.

WHAT IS LUPUS?

To put it simply, lupus is a condition whereby a person's immune system is in overdrive. It isn't cancer. It isn't AIDS—in fact, it's the exact opposite of AIDS. It isn't contagious. It's a chronic autoimmune disorder. Under normal conditions, the immune system functions to fight off viruses, bacteria, and germs by producing antibodies. In a person with lupus, the body cannot tell the difference between these foreign invaders and the body's healthy tissues. The body produces antibodies that attack healthy tissue. As some medical professionals put it, the body becomes allergic to itself.

"Lupus" is, of course, the Latin word for "wolf." The name could have been applied to the disease because the "butterfly rash" often associated with it was said to resemble the facial markings of a wolf.

According to the National Resource Center on Lupus, more than 16,000 new cases of the disease are reported annually across the country. The center estimates that at least 1.5 million Americans have lupus, but the actual number may be higher. Lupus can strike anyone, but it is most prevalent in women of childbearing age. It most commonly occurs in people between the ages of 15 and 44. "Women of color are two to three times more likely to develop lupus than Caucasians," the center reports.

The most common form of the disease is systemic lupus. It can affect the kidneys and is called lupus nephritis. Lupus can affect the brain and nervous system, and it can affect the heart.

Cutaneous lupus erythematosus is another form. It manifests itself in the skin and can cause a red and scaly discoid rash. Some patients suffer from the butterfly rash across the nose and cheeks.

According to the Mayo Clinic, "Some people are born with a tendency toward developing lupus, which may be triggered by infections, certain drugs or even sunlight. While there's no cure for lupus, treatments can help control symptoms." The clinic lists these symptoms:

- Fatigue and fever
- Joint pain, stiffness, and swelling
- Butterfly-shaped rash on the face that covers the cheeks and bridge of the nose
- Skin lesions that appear or worsen with sun exposure (photosensitivity)

- Fingers and toes that turn white or blue when exposed to cold or during stressful periods, known as Raynaud's phenomenon
- Shortness of breath
- Chest pain
- Dry eyes
- Headaches, confusion, and memory loss

In *The Lupus Book: A Guide for Patients and Their Families,* Dr. Daniel J. Wallace writes, "Lupus results when a specific predisposing set of genes is exposed to the right combination of environmental elements, infectious agents, lupus-inducing drugs, excessive ultraviolet light, physical trauma, emotional stress, or other factors."

According to the Lupus Foundation of America, 40 percent of adults with lupus and as many as 66 percent of all children with lupus will develop kidney complications. People with lupus take, on average, nearly eight prescription medications to manage all of their medical conditions, including lupus.

Although the disease is not curable, the Lupus Foundation estimates that some 80 to 90 percent of people who have lupus can expect to live a normal life span if their condition is closely monitored and medically treated. Lupus flares can be triggered by many factors, including stress, lack of rest, and overexposure to the sun.

4

THINKING BACK

—— JILL ——

As I read more and more about lupus, I learned that infection and sun exposure can trigger the disease. With that in mind, I began to look back on my life's events. It was 1959 when my family and I took the trip to Daytona Beach, Florida. The kind of sunscreen products so readily available today were virtually unheard of back then. We used Coppertone suntan lotion.

I had never been exposed to the sun to any great degree at age 3. We stayed in a duplex and had to walk to the beach. We took everything with us to spend the entire day on the beach. When we came in that evening, I was red all over and had broken out in blisters. My mother drew a cold-water bath for me and doused me in Solarcaine. From that point on, we knew that I didn't have the kind of skin that would tan. I tried to tan as a teenager, but within fifteen to twenty minutes, I would be blistered.

4-H was an important part of my life, beginning in fifth grade. I took part and won awards in home demonstration work, talent shows, and public speaking. I was president of the Scott County 4-H clubs my freshman year in high school, 1970 to 1971. When I was a sophomore, the county extension agent nominated me to become a Virginia State 4-H All-Star. I attended 4-H Congress at Virginia Tech in Blacksburg and after a week of activities was supposed to stay over the weekend and be inducted into the All-Star Hall of Fame. That ceremony was scheduled for Sunday. This was in June, but it was a chilly June. The temperature that week never got above 55 degrees, and it rained all week long. Expecting summer weather, all I took with me were shorts and tops, my Sunday dress outfit, and a light rain jacket.

In walking to the week's activities, I got wet and I got cold. I started feeling bad on Thursday evening. Everyone else was to leave on Friday except for the All-Stars. But I felt so bad that I rode the bus home with everyone else. I knew I was really sick. I had to miss the induction ceremony.

After returning home, I had a fever of 103 degrees. When I would lie down and try to raise up, I had excruciating pain in my chest but no cough or sinus drainage. My father took me to the emergency room at Holston Valley in Kingsport, where I was diagnosed with pneumonia. I suspect now that it was probably lupus pneumonitis.

My father made me an elixir of whiskey, honey, and lemon juice, and I would take a teaspoon of it every four hours. That loosened the congestion in my lungs so that I could finally cough.

I recovered from pneumonia but started having sinus infections. During my junior year in high school, I had five of them. Up until that bout with pneumonia, I had never missed a day of school since third grade. During the late months of 1972 and continuing through early 1974, I experienced repeated cases of sinus infections and sinusitis. With each case, I ran temperatures ranging from 100.5 to 101.5.

Dr. Miller always prescribed sulfa drugs along with an antibiotic each time I had a sinus infection. I would try to take the sulfa drugs but would experience extreme nausea. I would discover later that many lupus patients cannot take sulfa drugs.

My senior year, I felt better— good enough, in fact, to join the band and become captain of the flag corps. In August, before football season, we were out in the sun practicing every day. Because of the heat, we were given salt pills so that we would retain body fluid and not pass out with dehydration. I'm sure this had a harmful effect on my kidneys as well.

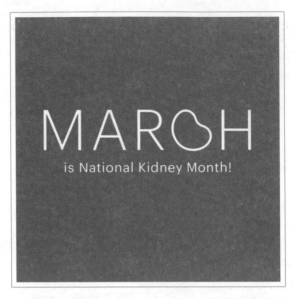

We hope this book will increase awareness of the vital role that
kidneys play in keeping us alive. Source: National Kidney Foundation.

When school started, band practice would take place after
school from 3:00 until 5:00 every day. I did not drink fluids from
the time I left to go to school until after 5:00, when I returned
home. Honestly, the reason was the fact that I did not want to use
the restrooms at my high school. I felt that they were unclean, and
there were no doors on the stalls. I was too modest to use them. All
I usually had in the morning was a small glass of milk. I truly feel
that these were among the reasons that lupus targeted my kidneys.

I seemed to get through my senior year in high school just
fine. I don't really remember being sick that year, just tired occasionally. That spring, the Gate City High School Marching Band
was the featured band at Disney World in Orlando, Florida. While
we were there, we spent time on the beach, in the sun.

I graduated from Gate City High School in May of 1974, fifth in
my class and ready to pursue a career in nursing. Soon after, I first
noticed the discoloration of my urine. I thought, "That's odd," and

hoped it would go away. On that mosquito-ridden trip to Myrtle Beach, I was exposed to the sun again.

Infections, sun exposure. Two of the conditions that bring on lupus converged. And I may also have been genetically predisposed for the disease since my maternal grandmother had died at such a young age.

5

A DREAM DENIED

—— JILL ——

I began my studies at East Tennessee State University in March of 1975 full of optimism about my future as a nurse, despite the setbacks that had come my way. I finished the spring quarter successfully and went back to Scott County for what I hoped would be a restful, uneventful summer. During the latter part of the summer, as I was preparing to return to college, I began to feel a slight twinge of pain in my right hip joint. By late fall, the pain was becoming more severe, and my left hip had begun to hurt as well. Still, I was determined to make it through the four-year nursing program. I asked my doctor that winter for some pain medication that wouldn't make me sleepy or drowsy. He prescribed Equagesic, which seemed to do the trick—at least at first.

On April 4, 1976, I was admitted to the hospital for an emergency appendectomy. I missed three weeks of school that quarter but was able to go back and finish with As and Bs. I had to take two incompletes but made up both of them later that summer.

The summer of 1976 seemed to provide a respite from my health problems. The protein count in my urine went down to a trace and then to zero. Dr. Miller reduced my Imuran dosage to 50 milligrams a day. Toward the end of that summer, after a twenty-four-hour creatinine clearance test, the dosage of Imuran was reduced yet again, to 25 milligrams a day.

But when I started back to college in September, my protein count quickly rose, to 3+ and 4+. We upped the Imuran to 50 milligrams again and then to 75, which kept the protein reading at 2+.

That fall, movement for me, except for plain walking, was getting increasingly difficult. There were days when I was very irritable, and I would cry because the pain in my hips was so bad. The Equagesic didn't help me any longer, but I kept pushing myself, trying to hide the fact that I was in constant pain. Some days I thought I was coming to my wits' end. The winter months were especially bad.

By the time I started my clinical training in nursing, in March of 1977, I was walking with a very noticeable limp. When I sat down and stood back up, I had to remain in place for a while before I could proceed to walk forward. I gritted my teeth with each step. The first two days of clinical training left me in bed for three days in pain.

It was time for a long talk with my nursing advisor and instructor, the late Dr. Shirley Turkett. "Jill, a nurse walks twenty miles a day and is on her feet all the time," she told me. She said it was time that I faced reality. I went ahead and finished out the quarter, taking only the classroom part of the nursing program, just for my benefit. But my days as a nursing major were over. My dream of becoming a nurse was dashed.

Through my first two years of college, I somehow managed to maintain grade point averages above 3.6 on the 4.0 scale, despite the stress and pain. However, the limited movement affected me socially. I didn't date that much because guys wanted to play tennis and the like, and I got tired of explaining my situation to them. It even bothered me to sit for two hours in a movie theater.

I decided to attend summer school that year to make up the hours that I had dropped. During the first part of the summer, I had to rely on crutches to get around, especially on days when it rained.

When the pain became intolerable, I came home after the first session of summer school and made an appointment with my doctor. He referred me to an orthopedist in Kingsport, Dr. Joseph Maloy.

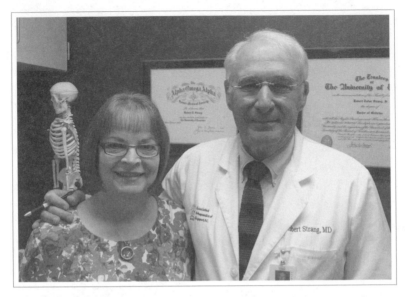

Dr. Robert T. Strang, Jr., performed one of Jill's hip replacement surgeries as well as hip surgery on Fred. Photo by Fred Sauceman

A new, previously unknown term to me was thus added to my vocabulary: aseptic necrosis. The high steroid doses, in the form of prednisone, had damaged my hip joints. The femoral head in the right hip was severely deteriorated, and the acetabulum had crumbled out. Dr. Maloy decided that a total hip replacement was necessary. At the time, I believe I was the youngest person ever to undergo that procedure at Holston Valley Community Hospital in Kingsport. At no point did I ever consider going outside the area for the surgery. Dr. Maloy was one of the best in the country, and I trusted him completely. The surgery was performed on August 10, 1977. The techniques and the technology for total hip replacements were far different in 1977 than they are now. Whereas now hospital stays last only a few days, I was hospitalized for two weeks.

Cement was used at that time to keep the prosthesis in place—both in the socket and around the shaft that was inserted into the leg. The cement had to solidify before I could put any weight on that leg. For older patients, doctors usually popped the hip joint out of place in order to perform the surgery, but since I was younger and my muscles and tendons were stronger, they had to cut through the muscle to dislocate the joint.

I was in bed, flat on my back, for three days after the operation. Nurses then got me up to sit on the side of the bed. The next day I was taken to physical therapy, still flat on my back. There, I was placed on a tilt board, which raised me up slowly to a standing position. Once I was in that position, they returned me to a reclining position and taught me leg exercises to strengthen the muscles around the joint. Slowly I was allowed to take a few steps with crutches.

After that first session, I could sit up without the help of the tilt board. I repeated this routine every day for the next week and a half. Soon I was able to negotiate steps.

After those two weeks, I was discharged. Whereas most patients had to have in-home therapy, the doctor trusted that I would do my exercises on my own. Within four weeks, I was driving again, but I had to remain out of school that fall.

"After you came home from the hospital from having your first hip replacement, I asked Angela Swiger [our neighbor then] to come sit with you and feed you lunch during the day since I was working at the elementary school," my mother remembers. "For doing that, I gave her all your nursing books and your uniforms since she was starting her clinical training in nursing that fall."

I reentered ETSU for the winter quarter of 1978 and was thinking about a career in music therapy since a nursing job on my feet would have significantly shortened the life of the prosthesis. The music therapy option would have required finishing at ETSU and then selecting another university for a master's degree. Because of the time that would take, I became concerned about finances since the Basic Educational Opportunity Grant only paid for four years. I took some courses in music theory but began to think about another career path.

I figured out that I could obtain a degree in community health education with a minor in psychology within that time frame if I went to summer school. BEOG did not pay for summer school, but my mother used the money she had earned as a teacher's aide at Hiltons Elementary School to send me to summer school in 1978.

In the spring of 1979, I graduated from ETSU with my BS in community health education. Knowing that I would soon be searching for employment, I decided to have the left hip replaced, even though it had not deteriorated quite as badly as the right one. In June of 1979, Dr. Maloy replaced the second hip. That time, I was only in the hospital ten days. I was still flat on my back for three days, but I had done so well with the first hip that I knew what to expect, and I had a good hip to rely on, thanks to the previous replacement.

During my recuperation period, Dr. Miller, in order to help me pay off some of my medical expenses, allowed me to come and work for his medical practice. I did medical transcription, and I worked with the health educator, who was a nurse.

6

"DATE HER YES, MARRY HER NO!"

—— FRED ——

This was the story Jill related to me that night on the ETSU campus. Admittedly, it was a lot to absorb. I believe it was probably the first time I had ever heard the word "lupus." And I knew very little about joint replacement surgery. What amazed me the most about everything she told me was how well she had kept her story hidden. She had suffered terribly for the preceding five years or so, but she masked the evidence with great skill and composure.

During our late-night conversation, she also told me that because of her condition, having children was pretty much out of the question. At that time, I was contemplating a career in television, which would have required a lot of moving around. With an unsettled, peripatetic life as a television news person likely ahead of me, I had thought very little about becoming a father. I also began immediately to think of my aunt, Mary Nelle Graves, a person I greatly admired who had led a very fulfilling life with no children of her own. I never heard her utter any words of regret about not being a mother. I would think of her often in the weeks and months ahead.

Hearing Jill's story did not change what I had originally told her. I did love her. Ending our relationship never entered my mind. In addition to confirming that love, her story deepened my respect and admiration for her. Other than some earaches and a tonsillectomy, I had led a healthy life. The specter of my father's brain cancer was always with me, but I worried very little then about health issues.

"I love you," I said again after our talk. This time, she said it, too.

My parents always thought I would marry a Greeneville girl. My mother and father, of course, didn't believe in arranged marriages as they are done in some cultures. But they had picked out a girl they hoped would be a future wife for me when I was in the first grade. I, however, always thought my marriage would result from a chance meeting with someone. For whatever reason, I always felt I would never marry a person I grew up around. In high school, the two girls I had dated the longest did not attend my high school. Both those relationships started with chance meetings.

In addition to her reaction when I had been out until after 4:00 in the morning with Jill, my mother questioned why I would want to marry someone from out of state. From the beginning, I had to defend my decision to date Jill.

Then, when I shared Jill's medical history with my mother, she began a campaign to dissuade me from marrying her. Just as I was unfamiliar with lupus, so was my mother. Without my knowing it, she met with our family doctor to get his advice. "Date her yes, marry her no!" was his admonition. That would become a mantra for my mother. I know that the doctor, who had delivered me, was looking out for what he thought was my best interest, but it's still difficult to imagine a health-care professional making such a comment. It stiffened my resolve to stay in the relationship.

East Tennessee State University has always been a very special place for us. One November afternoon, we were sitting on a bench in one of the loveliest spots on the campus, between Gilbreath Hall, an original campus building from 1911, and the Charles C. Sherrod Library. That's where I proposed marriage.

It was to be a long engagement, however. On that we both agreed. I was in my first quarter of graduate school, and we felt that I should complete my master's degree first. That would be almost two years. And Jill was facing her second total hip replacement

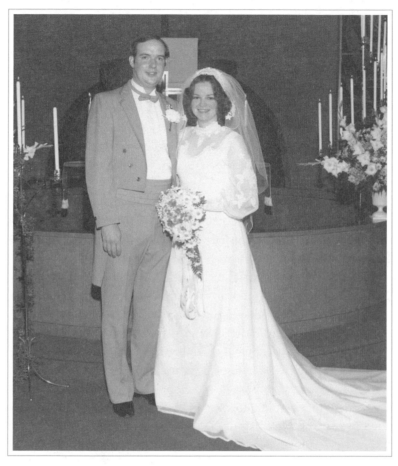

Our wedding, September 6, 1980. Photo by Ken Perry.

the next year. I gave her an engagement ring at Christmas in 1978. From initial meeting until official engagement, fewer than three months had passed.

In 1980, ETSU was converting from the quarter system to the semester system. Many of us in graduate school at that time accelerated our courses of study so that we would not run the risk of losing credit hours. While taking courses on the novels of William

Faulkner, the plays and poetry of T. S. Eliot, and a class called "The Legacy of Transcendentalism," that summer I had begun to work in the art department for American Greetings Corporation, at the company's Plus Mark facility in my hometown of Greeneville, Tennessee. I wrote copy for a new character called Strawberry Shortcake and her friends. I wrote copy for the company's catalogues. And I wrote copy for product packaging—boxed cards, gift wrap, and ribbons and bows. It was my mother's hope that I would land a permanent job there and settle in Greeneville, in one of the houses we owned.

My job with American Greetings was fascinating. I learned a great deal about design and printing that would serve me well as my career progressed. That part-time job also convinced me that an industrial setting was probably not ideal for me.

With marriage in my future and no solid prospects for permanent employment, I began to consider a military career. In the summer of 1980 I traveled to Knoxville to take the examination for Officers Candidate School in the United States Air Force. Although the test was heavily weighted toward mathematics and I had been away from calculus, algebra, and geometry for years, I somehow managed to pass it. My hope was to be selected for an assignment that would allow me to build on the skills I had developed in radio and television. When the assignment came, though, it wasn't even close. "Air Weapons Director" was my assigned role with the Air Force.

Meanwhile, I had gone to visit a family friend for advice. I had made the decision not to pursue a television career because of the nomadic life it would likely require. John M. Jones Sr. was the publisher of my hometown newspaper, *The Greeneville Sun*, then one of the finest small-town newspapers in the country. Mr. Jones was one of Greeneville's most influential and most well-connected people, and he was quite familiar with my work and with my family. In addition, he had statewide connections in education, having served for several years as chairman of the Tennessee Higher Education Commission.

A few weeks after that meeting with Mr. Jones, he called me to tell me that he had seen an old friend at a conference and had mentioned my name. That friend was Dr. Cuyler A. Dunbar, president of Roane State Community College in Harriman, Tennessee. Another chance meeting would change the course of my life. Dr. Dunbar told Mr. Jones that the college had a couple of openings. I immediately applied and was interviewed. Dr. Dunbar gave me a choice. I could take a faculty appointment in the college's Division of Humanities teaching English, or I could take an administrative position in the Office of Community Relations. I chose the public relations position since it would make heavy use of my media background. The job was ideal for me, combining my love of higher education with my love of radio, television, and newspaper work.

I turned down the Air Force, received my Master of Arts degree in English from ETSU, and started my new job at Roanc State—all within the course of a month. On September 5, 1980, I drove from Roane County, Tennessee, to Scott County, Virginia, for our rehearsal dinner. I remember doing a complete change of clothes while driving alone on Interstate 40. Ingrid Pfeiffer Carter catered the dinner for us, preparing a complete meal as she would have served it in her native Germany.

On September 6, Jill and I got married at Holston View United Methodist Church in Weber City, Virginia. After a reception at the church and another one back in Johnson City in the beloved Apartment 24, where I had lived during graduate school with my Greeneville buddies, Jill and I set out for Chattanooga, ultimately bound for a honeymoon in New Orleans.

"Date her yes, marry her no!" I had defied the directive. And I've never regretted it.

7

LUPUS REDUX

—— JILL ——

Our first house was a fully furnished one in Rockwood, Tennessee. As newlyweds, though, we were drawn to the active nightlife of Knoxville and took an apartment there in the spring of 1981. It was an exciting time to live in Knoxville, as the city hosted the 1982 World's Fair. Fred commuted back and forth to Roane State, and I found employment there as well. Through a Comprehensive Employment Training Act grant, I offered pre-employment training classes to inmates at Brushy Mountain State Penitentiary in Petros, Tennessee, at the Morgan County Regional Correctional Facility, and at Knox County Work Release. I taught them how to write a résumé, how to apply for a job, and how to handle a job interview. While I was teaching at Brushy, a sit-down strike over visitation privileges occurred among inmates, but I was unharmed.

Later, I worked as campaign associate for the Greater Knoxville Area United Way and through that position was able to land a job doing high blood pressure education and prevention activities in the public schools for the National Kidney Foundation of East Tennessee.

My activity level was high, and I felt reasonably good, although I did have a few periods of hypertension. One of Fred's responsibilities at Roane State was handling sports information for the school's athletic programs. I went on most of the road trips with the teams, and during home games, I even learned how to run the shot clock. We eventually moved back to Roane County—this time to Kingston—as our involvement with Roane State deepened.

Meanwhile, I knew that the Imuran I was taking to keep lupus under control could cause birth defects. I wanted to know what the options were if I accidentally got pregnant. Since my lupus had essentially been in remission for eight years, my gynecologist in Oak Ridge thought that perhaps I should discontinue the drug. But before taking me off the Imuran, he wanted the opinion of a nephrologist.

Dr. Ron Sinicrope admitted me to the Methodist Medical Center of Oak Ridge for a kidney biopsy. It showed almost normal kidney function with no lupus activity. However, some scar tissue was evident. The doctors concluded that I could come off the Imuran, thus alleviating any fear of having a child with a birth defect.

I was able to tackle two part-time jobs, one as a dental assistant and one as a social worker for VIP Home Nursing, both in Harriman. In Rockwood, Knoxville, and Kingston, we always rented, knowing that Fred would likely make a career move before too long. In 1984, the president of East Tennessee State University contacted Fred and asked him if he would be interested in heading up the university relations office at our alma mater.

Fred initially turned him down. Strangely, it was one of his hips that temporarily held him back. He had been experiencing leg pain while swimming and decided to have it checked out by an orthopedist from the group I had been seeing in Kingsport. When Dr. Robert Strang Jr. performed a biopsy, he found a hole in the leg as large as two eggs. Dr. Strang diagnosed it as a cartilage tumor in the right greater trochanter. He researched the case extensively before performing a bone graft in July of 1984. Fred was on crutches for nine weeks. Although Dr. Strang told Fred there was a 50-50 chance that the surgery would be effective, the graft worked perfectly.

In 1985, the president of ETSU called Fred again. By that time, he had been at Roane State for five years and was ready for a change. That summer, he assumed leadership of ETSU's alumni office and later added the university relations office to his list of responsibilities. Many of the faculty members who taught us at ETSU were

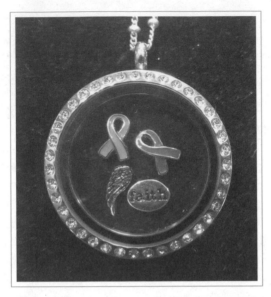

The locket Tina Graham made at a crucial time. Photo by Jill Sauceman.

still on campus, and it brought Fred a great deal of joy to be able to share their stories and promote their work. I secured a part-time job keeping the books for Volunteer Johnson City and, when time allowed, I volunteered as a tour guide, introducing travelers to the rich history of Jonesborough.

Before we left Roane County, I had begun to feel pain in my right hip, even when I was sitting. After we moved to Johnson City, I returned to Associated Orthopedics in Kingsport for an evaluation. The doctors discovered that the acetabular cup in my hip had shifted. The cement that had held it in was crumbling. This condition was likely brought on or at least worsened by the fact that I had taken part in a vocal and dance ensemble called The University Singers when I was a senior in college. I put up with the pain as long as I could, and when I could not tolerate it anymore, I asked my doctors to have the hip revised. Dr. Robert Strang Jr. and Dr. Maloy performed that surgery in July of 1988.

This time, instead of using cement, the surgeons employed a prosthetic material that bone would grow onto. Bone from the bone bank was placed in the socket, and I couldn't put full weight on my leg for two or three months, so that the bone would solidify and hold the acetabular cup in place. In surgery, the doctors had inserted two screws through the cup and into my pelvic girdle to keep everything in place until the grafted bone was firm. I remember going to Indian Rocks Beach in Florida that September and walking in the sand to rebuild muscle strength in my leg.

Doing bookkeeping work at Volunteer Johnson City inspired me to go back to school. I enrolled in the Master of Accountancy program at ETSU in 1989. Since I had taken no business courses as an undergraduate, my course load was heavy as I filled some gaps in my education. While I took courses, I worked as a graduate assistant in the Department of Accountancy. Professors always called on me in class, because they knew I would have my homework done. I was often up studying until 3:00 in the morning.

On January 14, 1992, my father died unexpectedly. My life became even more demanding as I traveled back and forth to Virginia to take care of my mother's needs while continuing to take graduate-level accounting and business courses and fulfilling the duties of my graduate assistantship. As I mentioned, stress is one of the triggers that can incite lupus flare-ups, and I had a major one. It affected every muscle and joint in my body, and I was in severe pain. I was able to make it through the spring semester at ETSU, but I decided to withdraw since I knew I was in a major lupus flare and needed as much rest as possible. This flare would take three years to get under control. Adding to my stress level was a nasty presidential change at ETSU in 1991 that Fred had to navigate through.

I was still seeing Dr. Miller in Kingsport, but the pain in my shoulders and arms made it difficult to drive there. In September of 1992, I sought the advice of Dr. Paul E. Stanton Jr., then Vice President for Health Affairs and Dean of the Quillen College of Medicine at ETSU. Dr. Stanton, a dear family friend who would become

president of ETSU in 1997, referred me to Dr. J. Kelly Smith, a
highly respected internal medicine physician and a member of the
medical school faculty. Dr. Smith wanted to get my lupus under
control without my having to take prednisone since I had developed so many side effects. I saw him almost weekly, and he was
the one who first directed me to a rheumatologist for lupus treatment. Dr. Smith also thought it advisable for me to begin seeing
a nephrologist and connected me with Dr. Clifford Wiegand in
Johnson City. In November of 1992, my rheumatologist, Dr. James
Myers, started me on Plaquenil, a medication used to treat malaria
(which, by the way, my father had contracted during World War II
in the Pacific). It made me feel some better, and I was also taking
Naprosyn, a nonsteroidal anti-inflammatory drug. But the pain
persisted, and I would repeatedly have to go back on small dosages
of prednisone, for it seemed to be the only thing that would take
the pain away. I knew, though, that I could not stay on it permanently. My body had proven that years before.

In December, I started experiencing pain in the center of the
chest, which Dr. Smith diagnosed as costochondritis, an inflammation of the junctions where the upper ribs join with the cartilage that connects them to the breastbone. It was yet another man-
ifestation of lupus. Throughout this period, I was running a low-
grade fever of 99.4 to 99.8 degrees. My list of doctors continued to
increase. I had to begin seeing an ophthalmologist because one of
the side effects of taking Plaquenil is retinal damage.

From my diary, December 31, 1992, is this entry: "Arms, shoulders, neck, and hands are very painful in muscles. Still have slight
headache. Hurts also at base of skull. As morning progresses, pain
moves to legs and feet. By noon I feel awful and achy. Still waking
up with very bad sore throat. For last few weeks have had sores on
my tongue. Still hurts to take deep breath. My blood pressure is
140/90 and my temperature is 99.4."

Again from my diary, January 1, 1993: "Excruciating pain and
aching all over body. Can hardly move and I shuffle my feet when
I walk. Pain persists across chest. Pain is much worse in the afternoon and I'm crying with frustration. BP 140/90. Temp. 99.6."

January 2, 1993: "Woke up in severe pain all over again and it's hard to move. I'm so frustrated and can't stop crying. Joints and muscles worse than yesterday. Headache continues. Sore place on left side of tongue was so painful yesterday that it was hard to eat. I can hardly open my mouth to brush my teeth because my jaws hurt so badly. My fingers and wrists are swollen. Supposed to attend a ballgame, but did not have the strength and in too much pain to go. Temp. 100."

January 3, 1993: "The pain is worse than ever now. Temp 100.5. Throbbing, burning pain in every muscle and joint. I am in tears most of the time. It's hard to take a deep breath because of pain across chest. Headache and sore throat worse. Becoming nauseated. Called Dr. Smith. After much discussion, we decided to go back on a large dosage of prednisone and discontinue the Naprosyn. By bedtime, I felt like a different person. No pain at all and in good spirits."

January 4, 1993: "Haven't felt this good or had this much energy in several years. Can concentrate better—thoughts are more clear. Lots more happy and cheerful. No pain anywhere. Swelling going down in feet, ankles, and hands. No sore throat."

As this diary entry shows, prednisone is indeed a miracle drug, but one with potentially devastating downsides. It was a battle for the next two years as I reduced the prednisone and balanced it with other drugs that had less serious side effects. All four of the drugs were salicylates: Disalcid, Ecotrin, Zorprin, and Salsalate, the last being the one that brought the best results.

Interestingly, each time my estrogen level increased during the monthly cycle, I would have a lupus flare-up with all the predictable symptoms. Those flare-ups would last for about two weeks. For half the month I would be fine, and I would be sick for the other half. Unlike the Imuran I took earlier that brought lupus into remission, the medications I took during the 1990s just controlled my lupus flares, and I continued to have days of pain. Somehow, these lupus flares did not seem to cause further kidney damage.

In 1995, Dr. Myers left Rheumatology Associates and I came under the care of Dr. David Lurie, who got me off the prednisone and was able to control the lupus with Plaquenil and Salsalate. When a generic Plaquenil came on the market in the late 1990s, I tried it but immediately broke out in hives. My body was reacting to something in the base of the generic brand. Dr. Lurie took me off it and placed me back on Imuran.

In 2001, I started having severe chest pains. Doctors attributed it to lupus, but it would happen right before I would start my menstrual cycle, and then it would go away. The pain recurred every month. It was hard for me to get my breath at night and turn over in bed. For a couple of years, I got very little sleep.

My wonderful primary care physician, Dr. J. Kelly Smith, retired in 2002. I had spent the past ten years with him. Knowing how important a doctor-patient relationship is to a lupus patient's well-being, he gave me his home telephone number, just in case I was ever in pain and needed him. But I didn't want to abuse this privilege, so I hardly ever called him during those ten years. He would chide me for not calling, since a call could have allowed him to help me sooner.

In the fall of 2003, I started experiencing extreme nausea, and my blood pressure was climbing. I managed to get through Christmas, but by New Year's Day, I was vomiting and my blood pressure was 200/100 and higher. Dr. Wiegand had been monitoring my kidney function, and my creatinine reading had been good, at around 0.9. As was the case throughout my battle with lupus, my kidneys were throwing off protein, and the reading was usually around 3+.

On January 2, 2004, I called Dr. Wiegand and told him how sick I was and how high my blood pressure had gotten. He instructed me to come to the office the very next morning. When he took my blood pressure, it was 232/134. He sent me straight to Johnson City Medical Center Hospital for admission. While there, I couldn't eat, and I continued to be nauseated. The doctors under whose care I was then placed tried all kinds of blood pressure medicines to try to get my blood pressure down. They decided that a CT scan of my lungs was needed, fearing that I had blood clots. I told them at the time that I didn't think blood clots were the problem, that I had been having the pain for three years, and that it came and went with my menstrual cycle. Because I once reacted to the contrast dye used in CT scans, the doctors ended up performing a VQ scan, which, I understand, is less accurate than a CT. The doctors said the scan showed what could be blood clots, and they placed me on Heparin, hoping that the blood-thinning medication would take care of the possible clots.

Every day I was in the hospital, it seemed, doctors would add another blood pressure medication. At one point I was taking eight different blood pressure drugs. The lowest my blood pressure got during that period was 180/100. I had been in the hospital for about three weeks when Dr. Wiegand recommended a kidney biopsy since my creatinine had risen. He wanted to make sure that if this was a lupus flare, the high blood pressure and lupus were not damaging my kidneys. At the time, most of the doctors coming in and out of my room felt I was experiencing a lupus flare.

Before a kidney biopsy could be performed without risking my health, my blood pressure needed to be lower than 150/90. Doctors decided to try me on a blood pressure medication called Norvasc. After I had taken the eight different blood pressure medications that had no effect, that one pill brought my reading down to 145/88. Once my blood pressure had dropped to that level, doctors believed it was safe to perform the kidney biopsy. The day arrived for the procedure, and I was taken to radiology. As in prior biopsies, I was placed on the CT table on my stomach with sand bags underneath. The radiologist used the CT scanner to locate the position of the kidney.

All of a sudden there was a lot of commotion in the room, and I had no idea what was going on. People were talking, and I heard one person say, "We've got to hurry up and get this done—get her off the table." Quickly, the radiologist inserted the needle, got his sample, and sent me back up to the room. As I was waiting on transport, I saw a person hooked up to several machines being wheeled in behind me. In the *Johnson City Press* newspaper the next day, I read about a terrible car accident involving a prominent local doctor who had been severely injured. That was the reason for the commotion in radiology. Only one CT scanner was working that day, and it was needed to ascertain the nature of the doctor's injuries.

I had to remain flat on my back for twenty-four hours to recover from the biopsy, which did show some lupus activity. While I was in the hospital, Dr. Lurie discussed with me the possibility of going on another immunosuppressive drug called Cellcept that might be more effective in protecting the kidneys.

Twenty-four hours after the kidney biopsy, the other doctors I was seeing in the hospital placed me back on Heparin, took me off the Norvasc, and put me back on all the other blood pressure medicines that I had been taking earlier. To this day, I cannot understand why that happened. I have chosen not to use those doctors' names in this book. The doctors who are the real heroes in this story are mentioned here by name.

Because there were so many cases of pneumonia on the floor where I was, doctors felt it best that I be discharged and go home. I was given prescriptions for all those blood pressure medicines and for Cellcept. I was also told that my blood was not thin enough, so the doctors sent me home with two Lovenox injections for the next two days, along with a prescription for Coumadin. I was instructed to go to my primary care doctor's office every day and get my blood checked until it was within the right levels.

I went on a Tuesday and had the test done. I was called that afternoon and told not to be around any knives or any sharp corners, that my blood was way too thin. I was to stop taking the Coumadin on Wednesday, resume taking it on Thursday, and get another blood test on Monday. I told the nurse my discharge orders indicated that I should get my blood checked every day until it reached safe levels. She said, "Oh, it'll be fine. Just do what I told you to do and come in Monday." It was far from fine.

8

"HELP ME, HELP ME!"

—— JILL ——

I gave the Cellcept a try, but it was making me nauseated. I had started it before I was discharged from the hospital and tolerated it well, but those were tablets. The only pharmacy then that had Cellcept available was Walgreens, and it only stocked capsules. In later research, I found that the capsule itself was made with sulfa— likely the reason for my nausea.

On Thursday, I resumed the Coumadin. On Saturday, I was at home writing thank-you notes to the people who had sent me cards and flowers and who had done kind things for me during my hospitalization. Fred had gone to Chilhowie, Virginia, to work on a magazine story. I got up to fix some chicken noodle soup for dinner and sat down at the table to eat it. Suddenly I was stricken with an excruciating pain in my side.

The first thing I thought of was that my kidney was bleeding from the biopsy site. Back when I had my first biopsy, I had some bleeding through the urine but no pain. When I got home from the hospital in Richmond then, I was told to place ice packs on my side, and within twenty-four hours, the bleeding was gone. When that pain hit me in Johnson City, I made an ice pack and went straight to bed to lie flat on my back with the ice pack placed on my side. The pain kept getting more intense, and I could hardly take a deep breath. I was within seconds of calling 911 when Fred called on his way back from Chilhowie to ask me if I needed anything from the grocery store.

"Where are you?" I asked. He told me he had just gotten into Johnson City. "Forget the grocery store," I said. "Get home as soon as possible. I need to go to the emergency room."

By the time Fred got in the door, I was barely able to put a jacket on and make it to the car. When we got to the emergency room, I couldn't walk. If I moved only slightly, the pain would take over my entire body. One of the patients who was at the ER for treatment helped Fred get me into a wheelchair. As soon as I got in the door, the staff wanted to ask me questions, but I was in too much pain to answer. I remember saying, "Help me, help me! I'm going to throw up!"

Staff members immediately rushed me into a nurse's office, where I got sick just from the sheer pain, I'm sure. The staff proceeded to ask me a series of questions for the required paperwork. I answered the best I could, but I just wanted someone to put me out of my misery.

I was eventually taken to a room on a gurney, and it seemed forever before anyone came to see me. I was rolling from side to side in misery. Fred kept leaving the room to try to find someone to help me.

Finally, several medical personnel arrived and attempted to start an IV, but they couldn't find a vein. I was severely dehydrated. Someone from Wings Air Rescue, a trauma specialist, was able to find a vein. As soon as that medicine hit me, I lost consciousness and did not regain it until Monday. One vague memory involved being placed onto a table for a CT scan, without contrast. That was all I recalled until Monday, when hospital staff were shaking me to try to get me awake.

I did indeed have a large hematoma in the abdomen, the result of a blood clot at the renal biopsy site having broken loose. My once extremely high blood pressure became so low that the medical personnel couldn't even get a reading.

Because I had been on blood thinner, surgery could not be performed to stop the bleeding from my kidney. I was given seven units of blood to replace my blood loss, along with large doses of

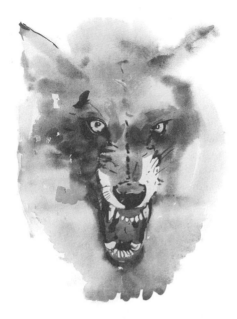

vitamin K to help my blood clot. At that point, it was a waiting game to determine if I could survive the trauma.

After I finally woke up on Monday, the hospital notified my primary care physician. When he saw me, his response was, "I guess I could have had you come in Friday instead of Monday." I just looked at him. I never saw him again as a patient. Again, his name is never mentioned in this book.

Dr. Wiegand, my steadfast nephrologist, was called in. He told me that he had reviewed the situation and that my creatinine reading, at 4.5, was half a point shy of dialysis and that he would keep monitoring my case to determine the direction we should take.

For a week, I had to lie flat on my back. Even the slightest move to turn me to change the bed still resulted in unbearable pain. After the bleeding subsided and the pain started easing off, I was able to sit up in bed.

With every IV and blood transfusion, I was given a bag of saline. Since my kidneys weren't functioning well, I was retaining all that fluid. I gained about forty pounds in fluid. By the third week, I was able to stand and move around some, but I was still on oxygen. Because of the extra weight, it was difficult for me to move.

As I recuperated, my blood pressure started to rise, to around 180/100, but my creatinine started to trend in the right direction. I was able to avoid dialysis, but barely. By the third week of my second hospitalization that winter, my creatinine was down to 2.5.

I had been in the hospital this time for almost four weeks. Together, my two hospital stays lasted for about two months. My blood pressure all through the month of March hovered around 180/100, and I was afraid to do too much because of the risk of a stroke or heart attack. By that time, I was taking six different medications to treat the blood pressure. I also had a touch of pneumonia in my lower left lung, a result of being in bed for so long. My creatinine was trending downward, but it would never reach my pre-hospitalization levels.

I was able to find Cellcept tablets instead of capsules and started on those. The drug helped preserve my kidney function while keeping the lupus under control.

At my appointment in April for a checkup with Dr. Wiegand, I expressed concern about my continued high blood pressure. I told him that none of the medications were working but that I had been given one medication in the hospital, for a total of about two days, that had brought my blood pressure down enough for the kidney biopsy to be performed. I told him I couldn't understand why those doctors did not leave me on that particular medicine. He then wrote me a prescription for Norvasc. I had it filled and took the medicine the next day. My blood pressure almost instantly came down to a safe level. Taking 10 milligrams of Norvasc, I recorded blood pressure readings of 130/80, which is fairly good for someone suffering from chronic kidney disease. I stopped all the other medications that had no effect on my blood pressure whatsoever.

It took me six months of recuperation before I could go back to work. In the interim, I began to work at home. My coworkers at the Heritage Alliance of Northeast Tennessee and Southwest Virginia moved my entire office into my home so that I could resume keeping the books for this nonprofit organization headquartered in Jonesborough, Tennessee. That was as therapeutic for me as any medicine. It kept my mind off my recurring nausea, and it helped me feel productive and useful again. I will be forever grateful to the organization for keeping a place for me and for going to these lengths to allow me to work again.

As for the nausea, I felt like my kidneys could not be the cause, for my creatinine was running around 1.4. Ultrasounds of my abdomen had been done during my hospitalization, and I was told that I did not have gallstones. By 2005, the nausea had worsened. One Saturday, I had gone to a local restaurant for a gravy biscuit and then to the home improvement store Lowe's. As I was standing in the checkout line, I was hit with a kind of abdominal pain that I had never experienced before. I made it home, got sick, and immediately felt better.

In late spring, our office went to a Mexican restaurant for lunch, which began with chips and salsa. I had another attack that evening with the same kind of abdominal pain. It was the same pattern—get sick, feel better.

At an appointment with Dr. Wiegand, my nephrologist, I asked him if a person could have gallbladder problems without having gallstones, since I was told I had no stones. He said that was most definitely possible and ordered a more thorough ultrasound of the abdomen, pancreas, and gallbladder.

I received a call at home a few days later from Dr. Wiegand, who told me that my gallbladder was "full of sludge." We made arrangements for me to have gallbladder surgery in September of 2005. The surgery was done laparoscopically. I was able to eat immediately afterward, and I did not take any pain medication. Within a week, I was back at work. Thinking back on it now, I believe that the gallbladder was my problem when I was initially hospitalized in 2004. Further, during my second hospitalization in 2004, when I was taken off the Coumadin, Dr. Lurie, my rheumatologist, had suspected that I actually had pulmonary endometriosis instead of blood clots in my lungs. I was never placed back on Coumadin. After going through menopause in 2008, I never had another chest pain. That confirmed his diagnosis.

In 2007, another kidney biopsy was performed at Johnson City Medical Center Hospital. Dr. Wiegand was troubled by the continued drop in my glomerular filtration rate (GFR). The biopsy indicated that the damage to the nephrons and glomeruli in the kidneys was irreversible. My best option at the time was to try to tolerate the drug Cellcept and its gastrointestinal side effects. Those side effects eventually became intolerable. I believe that because of my decreasing kidney function, the drug was becoming toxic to my system. We tried lowering the dosage by half. That worked for a while, but the Cellcept would build up in my system, causing constant diarrhea.

After discussing possible alternatives to Cellcept with both doctors, Lurie and Wiegand, I decided to go back on Imuran. The drug had helped me immensely after I was first diagnosed with lupus, but the kidney disease was too far advanced by 2010. It kept my lupus in remission, but it did not help my kidneys.

I had monthly blood work at Dr. Lurie's office but saw him only every six months since lupus was not giving me much trouble. My appointments with Dr. Wiegand occurred every two months. Around 2008, my kidney function had deteriorated to the point where my GFR was at 20. I was in stage 4 chronic kidney disease (CKD), described as a "severe loss of kidney function."

A patient can be evaluated for the kidney transplant list when the GFR reading hits 20 or below. I had always been told that if one could maintain a GFR of 20, a normal life was possible for years. My kidney function would fluctuate—going as low as 15 and then rising back to nearly 20. The hopes that Fred and I had for my future rose and fell repeatedly every month as those test results came back.

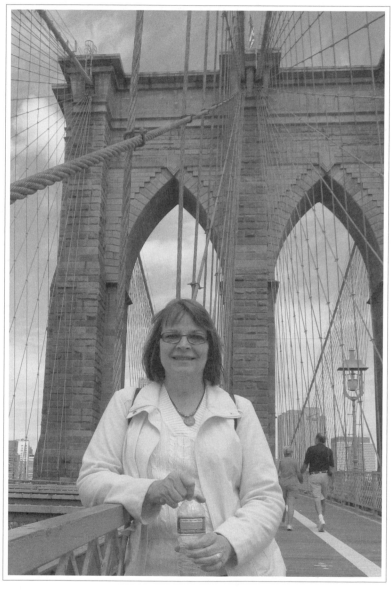

While Jill was in kidney failure, she managed to walk the Brooklyn Bridge.
Photo by Fred Sauceman.

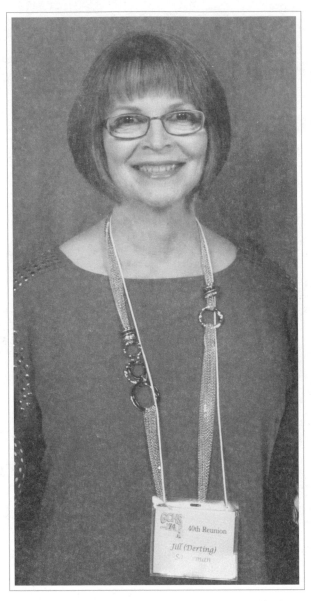

Despite being in kidney failure, Jill managed to plan her
40th high school reunion. Photo by Nathan Carter.

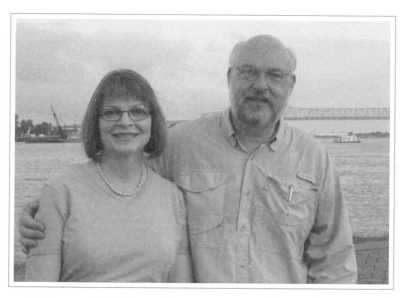

We honeymooned in New Orleans and have returned many times since.
Photo by Larry Smith.

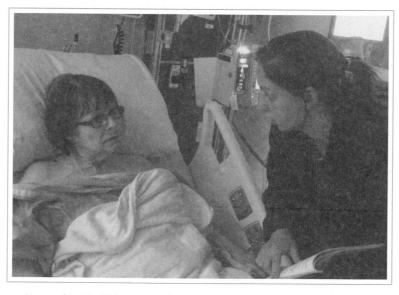

Hours after the kidney transplant surgery, nurse Jessica Walker provides
one-to-one care for Jill at Vanderbilt. Photo by Fred Sauceman.

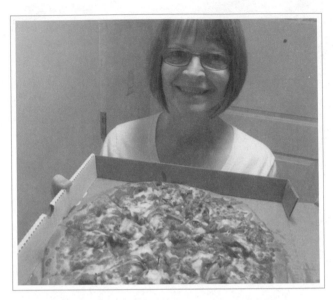

The doctor-recommended cheese pizza, plus a little more,
four days after the transplant. Photo by Fred Sauceman.

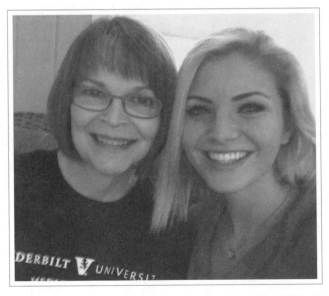

Olivia Caridi, then with WCYB-TV in Bristol, Virginia, shared Jill's kidney
transplant story with her viewers. Photo by Olivia Caridi.

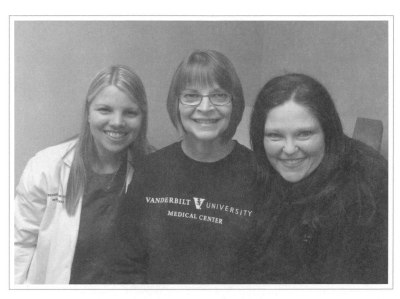

Two of the people who took care of Jill after her transplant, Kristin Smith, RN, and April DeMers, MSRN, ACNP-BC. Photo by Fred Sauceman.

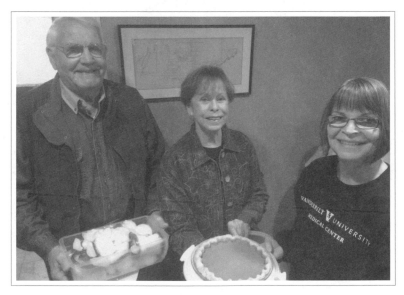

Glen and Dot Whittington brought homemade ice cream and pumpkin pie that unforgettable Thanksgiving Day in 2014. Photo by Fred Sauceman.

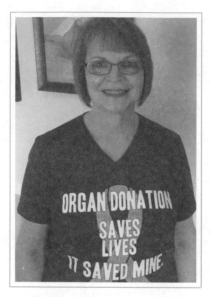

We have become passionate organ donation advocates.
Photo by Fred Sauceman.

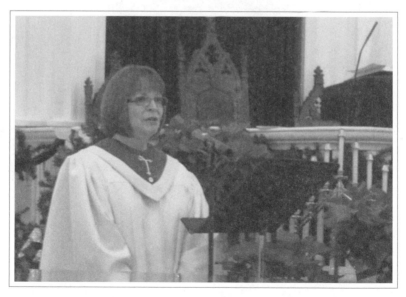

With a new kidney, Jill resumed singing at Jonesborough
Presbyterian Church in 2015. Photo by Fred Sauceman.

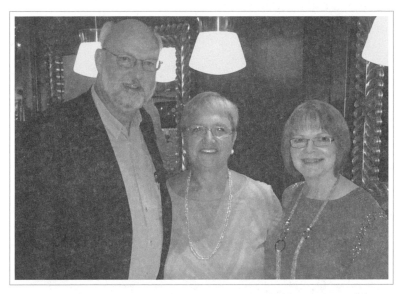

Our first return trip to New York City after Jill's transplant coincided
with our 35th wedding anniversary. We celebrated at Felidia
in Manhattan with famed food personality Lidia Bastianich.

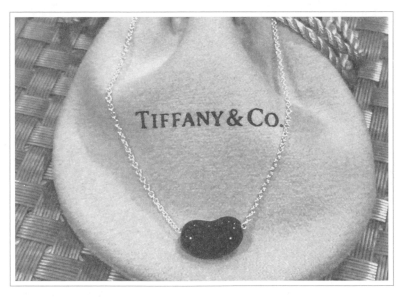

For a 35th wedding anniversary present, Fred gave Jill a black jade bean
necklace to represent her new kidney. Photo by Jill Sauceman.

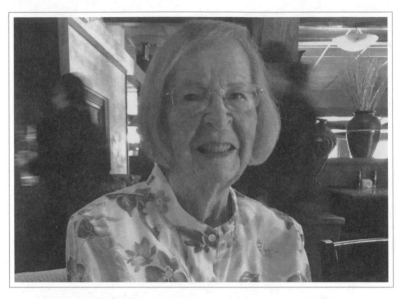

Jill's mother Elsie Derting, on her 94th birthday in 2017.
Photo by Jill Sauceman.

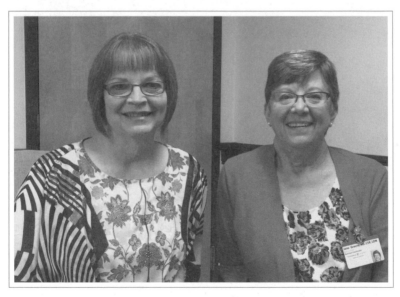

Vanderbilt renal transplant dietitian Jane Greene assists kidney patients
in developing healthy eating habits. Photo by Fred Sauceman.

9

"WHICH WAY IS RIGHT?"

—— FRED ——

As Jill's kidney disease worsened, my mother's mental and physical health began to decline. Before her retirement in 1993 at age 70, she had worked in the accounting department at Greene Valley Developmental Center in Greeneville, Tennessee. She had always been good with numbers. Before I was born, she ran the business operations of a dress factory, and after I had been in elementary school for a few years, she worked part-time for the Greeneville-Greene County United Fund (now the United Way) and later for the Austin Company, one of the world's largest tobacco dealers.

In 2006 she began calling Jill, the skilled bookkeeper, saying she could not balance her personal checkbook, despite the fact that typically no more than five checks had been written for the month. The telephone, cable, and gas bills were automatically drafted from her account. That gave her difficulty because she would receive statements before the money was taken out of the account. There would be marks and figures all over the checkbook and her statement, and Jill had to unravel what she had done.

Finally, in 2008, Jill convinced my mother to allow her to take over the checkbook balancing entirely. We noticed, too, that she had lost the ability to evaluate her mail and could not tell the difference between junk mail and legitimate mail. She had been donating to every charity imaginable.

My mother had also developed diabetic neuropathy, which caused numbness in her feet, but she continued to drive. On two occasions, she failed to stop her car in time and dislodged the wall of her garage. We constructed a barrier on the floor of the garage to keep such incidents from happening again.

In addition, my mother had a thyroid problem, which required trips to an endocrinologist in Bristol, and she was seeing an ophthalmologist and a podiatrist in Johnson City as well as her primary care physician and dentist in Greeneville. Managing her care was becoming a full-time job, and Jill, the person my mother had instructed me not to marry, became her caregiver. Jill left her job in 2008 in order to travel to Greeneville two and three days a week to attend to her needs. Being an only child has its distinct advantages, but in situations like this one, a brother or sister would have been a godsend.

When I was young, my mother and I visited relatives in nursing homes often. As she aged, she begged me never to go that route with her. Her ambition was to come and live with us in Johnson City, but with my job and Jill's health, that wasn't possible. This caused many painful and protracted arguments between my mother and me. "I'm going to come back and haunt you if you ever put me in a nursing home," she threatened often. In public, she would say to friends, "Jill and Fred don't want me."

My job at East Tennessee State University was an all-consuming one, and in 2008, the demands on my time increased even more when ETSU President Dr. Paul E. Stanton Jr. asked me to serve as chairman of the university's centennial celebration, which would culminate in 2011. Even with an ailing wife and a declining mother, I chose to accept. Given my long history with the university, I viewed it as the assignment of a lifetime.

My mother had largely lost her ability to cook and was not eating properly. We cooked food for her and delivered it to Greeneville, and several of her friends pitched in. For months, she had talked about trying to qualify for Meals on Wheels. She didn't qualify financially, so we paid for the service and never told her.

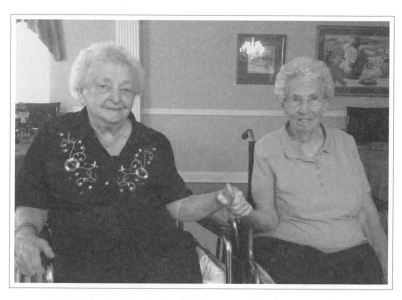

Fred's mother Wanda and her longtime friend Elsie Creamer.
Photo by Fred Sauceman.

That lasted a few months. Jill would visit her and find food in the refrigerator that people had brought her and Meals on Wheels servings left in the freezer. She had lost her ability to use the microwave and didn't trust herself with the stove or oven. She was picking up cookies and crackers off the kitchen counter, and that was the extent of her diet.

I had begun calling my mother every morning. She would say things like, "Where have you been?" She would tell me about her mother being there with her, although my grandmother had been dead since 1971. She began saying that she was seeing rats throughout the house and rats crawling across the bed. She would claim that someone had been beating on the house at night.

I remember visiting her one Saturday afternoon and finding her no longer able to check her blood sugar, which she had been doing faithfully for years. For two years afterward, Jill assembled her medicines to cover morning, noon, and night dosages for every month.

My mother soon forgot how to lock her doors. Jill placed sticky notes above every door lock with directions. "Which way is right?" my mother asked. She couldn't understand "turn to the right," so Jill had to draw arrows on each note to indicate how the key should be turned.

We discovered that she had begun to experience falls, especially at night when she would get out of bed. She would press her Medic Alert button, and emergency medical technicians would call one of her friends who had a key to the house. She tried to joke about her falls, including one she had in the parking lot of Doughty-Stevens Funeral Home.

Every year before Memorial Day, she would place flowers on the graves of my father and her sister at Oak Grove Cemetery in Greeneville. She became fearful that the flowers would be stolen and demanded that we come down and remove them the day after Memorial Day, which we were unable to do. We told her we would get them as soon as possible and warned her not to try to get them herself. She wouldn't listen.

On a 90-degree day, she went to the cemetery alone and fell. An engineer in a passing train spotted her, and a lady who lived near the cemetery took her home, after she had lain there for about two hours. On another occasion, she had arranged for a dental hygienist at her dentist's office to pick her up and take her to her routine appointment. She decided to walk down her driveway and wait on the hygienist's arrival. She lost her balance and fell straight backward, hitting her head on the pavement. Bleeding profusely from the head, she was taken by the hygienist to a local hospital. Miraculously, through all these falls, this woman nearing 90 years of age never suffered a broken bone.

On a visit to her primary care physician, we were able to sign my mother up for home health physical therapy to try to help with her instability. One afternoon, when Jill took her to a Greeneville pharmacy to fill a prescription, she was overcome with heat exhaustion. They sat in the pharmacy until my mother cooled off and Jill was able to get her home. Physical therapists from a home health agency came to her house. While they were there, she had another episode and wanted to go to bed. After the physical therapists left, she started writhing as if she were in pain, and she seemed disoriented. Jill pressed the Medic Alert button, and EMTs arrived. I left work to meet Jill and my mother at the hospital. She was examined, we were told nothing was wrong, and she was discharged.

We have always been "dog people." My mother had been around dogs all her life and continued that tradition into old age. As long as her Boston Bull Terrier was alive, she managed to function, but after the dog became infirm and had to be euthanized in March of 2011, her world started collapsing on her more rapidly. But Jill was able to bring her to ETSU when I delivered commencement speeches to the graduating class in May. It was the last time she ever made her famous potato rolls, a recipe inherited from her mother.

There were mishaps and falls all summer long as we struggled to figure out how to deal with this awful dilemma. The arguments about living arrangements intensified. We had taken my mother to visit two very nice facilities, Morning Pointe in Greeneville and Colonial Hills in Johnson City. She refused Morning Pointe, but somehow we got her to agree to be put on a waiting list for Colonial Hills, just a ten-minute drive from our house. We thought a home sitter might be a possibility. We found a lady and hired her, but my mother fired her within two days.

As all this was happening, the ETSU Centennial was in full swing, consuming my days and most of my evenings as we headed toward its culmination in October of 2011. At the same time, my food-writing career was taking off. One Saturday we had gone to Burnsville, North Carolina, where I spoke at a literary conference. We came home that evening exhausted and thinking about all that we were facing that fall. The telephone rang at 2:00 the next morning. Jill answered. It was an EMT from Greeneville, saying

that my mother had fallen again and that she was being transported to the hospital. "You need to do something about this situation," the EMT said. "This is the seventh time we've been to her
house in two weeks to get her up off of the floor."

When we arrived in Greeneville, doctors at the hospital kept
telling us they really couldn't find anything wrong. "This is an
88-year-old who has been falling repeatedly," I told the doctor in
charge of the emergency room that morning. "I'm not taking her
back home. You need to admit her to the hospital and figure out
what is causing these falls."

"Let me see what I can do," the doctor told us. She was admitted
to the hospital with the diagnosis "failure to thrive." By that point,
she was unable to walk. Once she got into a hospital room, she
was combative. She was there for three days. For the first day, she
thought she was at ETSU and that the doctors were professors and
the nurses students. The second day she claimed she was in a pris-
oner of war camp during World War II, being held captive by the
Nazis. On the third day, she thought she had been kidnapped by a
religious cult and had been taken to a church service.

Jill and I had begun meeting with a hospital social worker to
get her admitted to a rehabilitation facility so that she could start
walking again. We knew, down deep, that she would likely never
go home again.

Earlier that summer, I had contacted an old friend of mine, Dr.
Ron Hamdy, one of the top gerontologists in the world, who held
a faculty appointment with ETSU's Quillen College of Medicine.
Dr. Hamdy kindly agreed to evaluate my mother, and we got her
to Johnson City on the pretext of checking her balance. The real
purpose of the visit, though, was to determine if she had dementia.
She went through all the testing and then became furious. "Are you
trying to put me in a home?" she asked. In front of Dr. Hamdy, I
told her that with Jill's health problems, we could not take care
of her in our home. "You're no son of mine," she yelled. Then she
stormed out of Dr. Hamdy's office. I'm sure Dr. Hamdy had wit-
nessed much worse, but that was certainly a low point in my life.

Jill had to take my mother back to Greeneville, and she told me it was the longest, quietest ride of her life.

Through the help of that social worker in Greeneville, we were able to transfer my mother from the hospital to NHC Healthcare in Johnson City. She was to be there 100 days to take physical therapy and learn to walk again. She was placed in a double room but was combative with her roommate, so we were forced to move her to a private room. She was both physically and verbally abusive to us—especially to me, since she blamed me for what she felt was a type of incarceration. All the while she was at NHC that fall, she begged to go home. We told her a return home was impossible until she was able to walk again.

Dr. Hamdy diagnosed my mother with three forms of dementia—vascular, Alzheimer's, and primarily Lewy body dementia, another medical term we knew little about until that point. According to the Lewy Body Dementia Association, the disease affects some 1.4 million people and their families in the United States. Its symptoms closely resemble other more commonly known diseases such as Alzheimer's and Parkinson's. "Many doctors or other medical professionals still are not familiar with LBD," the association says. Among the symptoms are "recurrent complex visual hallucinations, typically well formed and detailed," and "repeated falls." Finally, through the knowledge of Dr. Hamdy, we had some answers.

The disease takes its name from the work of Dr. Friederich H. Lewy who, according to the association, "discovered abnormal protein deposits that disrupt the brain's normal functioning."

Dr. Hamdy prescribed the antipsychotic medication Risperdal (Risperidone), which did not eliminate the hallucinations entirely but drastically reduced them and made my mother far more pleasant to be around.

My mother responded well to the physical therapy and was able to walk up and down the halls of NHC with the help of a walker. She could even walk to the dining room and back, whereas before, she had to be transported by wheelchair.

By November of 2011, she was mobile enough for a lunchtime visit to the Olive Garden with Jill and me in Johnson City. With the help of NET TRANS vans that could accommodate wheelchairs, she returned to her dentist in Greeneville for a checkup and went to eye and ear-nose-and-throat appointments in Johnson City. By Christmas, we were able to bring her to our home for lunch.

My mother was never one to share compliments. When my aunt Zella Bible had died a few years earlier, I was selected to be a pallbearer. Immediately after the funeral service, my mother made a beeline for me, saying, "You know, you were the only one of those pallbearers whose hair wasn't tapered."

But that Christmas day in 2011, she told us both, "You all have done very well in life. I'm proud of you." My mother and I had come through some awful times. We had shared harsh words. We had ended many a visit abruptly, both at our home and hers. After all the conflict, those simple words of praise and reconciliation meant the world to me. She seemed to come to terms with all my life's decisions that she had questioned, including my choice of a wife. By late afternoon that Christmas day, this person who had so resisted life in a nursing home started looking at her watch to make sure she got back to NHC in time for dinner.

Once my mother's 100 days of therapy were over, she had progressed to the point where she was getting around well with a walker. Going home, though, was still out of the question, and she was moved to the long-term care wing at NHC in March of 2012.

By that time, Jill was in end-stage renal failure with a very low energy level. Nevertheless, she visited my mother at NHC three days a week, just like she had done in Greeneville. My mother was of the generation of women who were accustomed to having their hair done every week. NHC itself had a beauty shop, but Jill bought a portable hair dryer unit and would go every Friday morning to do my mother's hair. Visitors would compliment my mother on her hairstyle and would ask if Jill was a professional beautician. She had no training in cosmetology but had observed the techniques the hairdressers in Greeneville used and was able to copy them.

And Jill did my mother's laundry for more than two years. I relate so many details of my mother's decline to give a sense of the pressures we were dealing with as Jill's kidney disease advanced and to underscore the irony of Jill turning out to be my mother's primary caregiver, even though my mother had resisted and fought against our marriage so strongly.

Easter has always been a special time in my family, and we wanted my mother to share in the celebration that spring of 2012. We struggled to get her in and out of the car but made it into our house for Easter lunch. When it came time to take her back to NHC, we almost had to leave her in the driveway. She couldn't follow instructions to back up and get in the car seat and couldn't help us maneuver her in any way. While I held onto her to keep her off the ground, Jill got into the driver's seat and grasped her under her arms. While I shoved, Jill pulled, and we got her into the car seat. When we got back to NHC, we enlisted the help of the trained staff to get her out of the car and back to her room.

A few months later, I got a call late one afternoon from a staff member at NHC, who told me that my mother had tumbled forward out of her wheelchair onto the floor face first. Her face was terribly swollen, cut, and bruised. She was transported to the emergency room at Johnson City Medical Center, where she was x-rayed before returning to NHC that evening. Even at the age of 89, she suffered no broken bones from the fall out of the wheelchair.

On a Friday afternoon that September, Jill called me from the office of my mother's ophthalmologist. She had taken her to the bathroom, and it took all the strength Jill had to keep her from falling on the floor. She told me that she could no longer take her out of NHC without help.

That very day, I received an email from one of my employees at ETSU, Wayne Winkler, director of public radio station WETS-FM/HD, which was part of my division. Wayne told me in that email that he thought it was time for the station to hire a news person. While I loved my job, I was quickly coming to the conclusion that something had to change. With a mother in this condition and a wife at serious risk of dying from kidney failure, I had been running through possible employment scenarios in my mind. When I received that email from Wayne, I took it as a sign. I explained my situation to him and asked if he would consider me for the news job on a part-time basis. I had worked for the state for thirty-two years by that time and had qualified for full retirement two years earlier. Dr. Brian Noland, ETSU's president, generously worked out an arrangement allowing me to do news every day on WETS and to fill out the rest of my part-time employment contract by writing and doing public relations work for the office I had supervised since 1985. At the end of 2012, I gave up my dream job and became a part-time, temporary employee. I had come full circle, since my very first job in radio when I was 15 years old required me to deliver the news.

By 2013, my mother had lost all control of her legs. She was approved for two more weeks of therapy in a futile attempt to get her walking again. This lady who had enjoyed food so much throughout her lifetime had to be placed on a diet of thickened liquids and puréed food, since she could not swallow easily. On the days Jill went to NHC, she tried to arrive at lunchtime so she could feed my mother by hand. Even with insulin shots and pills, my mother's blood sugar remained out of control, hitting levels as high as 350 to 380. The year 2013 was a steady downward trek for her, but she was able to participate in her ninetieth birthday party on May 10 with a roomful of friends and family.

In March of 2014, during one of our regular patient care conferences, NHC staff told us it was time to bring in hospice. Death wasn't imminent, but my mother's case was clearly terminal. Caris Hospice took over her bathing and the administration of her medications.

Early in the morning of August 21, 2014, we received a call from a nurse at NHC indicating that my mother had taken a turn for the worse and that she could not eat or drink. The staff at NHC suspected that she had had another stroke. Hospice told us that day that she would likely pass away within a week. She made it through the night, and we returned to see her on Friday. She was unresponsive and was struggling to breathe. Around 4:00 the next morning, NHC staff came to check on her and discovered that she had died. I had prepared her obituary months before and simply had to fill in the details of her passing.

During her graveside service at Greeneville's Oak Grove Cemetery, Jill sang a duet with our friend Mary Lynn Lancaster. My mother had selected the song, "In the Garden," and had asked Jill to sing it.

I cannot imagine getting through the last years of my mother's life without Jill. Even though I know she often didn't feel like getting out of bed in the morning, she became my mother's guardian angel.

10

MAKING THE LIST

—— JILL ——

In the spring of 2013, my glomerular filtration rate never rose above 15. Dr. Wiegand told me, "I think now is the time when I should refer you to be evaluated for the kidney transplant list, wherever you choose to go." He mentioned the University of Virginia in Charlottesville, the University of Tennessee in Knoxville, Duke University in Durham, North Carolina, and Vanderbilt University in Nashville, Tennessee. I had already made up my mind that Vanderbilt University Medical Center was the place where I wanted to go.

Kidney patients can be referred for evaluation for the transplant list at a GFR of 20 or below. I had spent the last four years in that range but had adjusted to the decreased kidney function so well that Dr. Wiegand delayed discussing transplantation for as long as he could. When my GFR reached 15, though, he said, "I wouldn't be carrying out my responsibilities as your doctor if I didn't go ahead and refer you."

Dr. Wiegand sent a letter and copies of my files to the Kidney/ Pancreas Transplant Program at Vanderbilt, and I was contacted for an evaluation appointment in August. Before I went to Nashville, Dr. Wiegand referred me to a local dialysis center in Johnson City, where I met with a social worker to talk about the various forms of dialysis. Because of that visit, I made the decision to prepare myself for peritoneal dialysis. It's a form of dialysis that filters the blood using the peritoneum, the lining of the cavity that surrounds the organs in the abdomen. It uses a special cleansing solution that flows from a bag through a catheter and into the stomach. This kind of dialysis can be performed at home. It's done seven days a week for eight to ten hours a day. Most patients dialyze themselves while they sleep. I chose this option over hemodialysis, which is done only three days a week. I was fearful that after having lupus for so many years, my blood vessels might not withstand hemodialysis. I thought, too, that peritoneal dialysis might be easier to administer while we traveled.

Dr. Wiegand decided to leave it up to me to tell him when my symptoms got so severe that dialysis was inevitable. He instructed me to give him at least two weeks' notice so that a catheter could be surgically inserted in my abdomen. That incision would need time to heal before peritoneal dialysis could begin.

August 14, my first day of evaluation at Vanderbilt, began around a meeting room table with several other kidney patients and their families. I remember the bulging bags of medication that the other patients had brought with them. I was on four different medicines at the time.

One of those patients we would come to know and follow over the ensuing months. His name was Julius Blevins. We became instantly interested in his story because he and his wife, Diana, were from Saltville, Virginia, in the southwestern part of the state, not too far from where I grew up. Julius suffered from PKD—polycystic kidney disease. One of his kidneys was removed at Bristol Regional Medical Center some time after our first meeting because it had become so diseased. On one of our later encounters at Vanderbilt, Diana showed us a picture of that kidney. A normal kidney weighs about five or six pounds. His weighed eighteen. When Julius came to that August meeting, he had already lined up a live donor. Our families came to support each other and cheer each other on through the power of social media.

The day of the evaluation consisted of nonstop appointments, beginning with a patient education session on kidney transplantation, a meeting with a social worker, and a series of

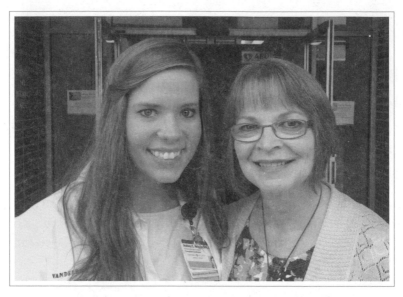

Ashley Wilson, RN, was one of Jill's nurses on 7th Floor Critical Care and is
now a transplant coordinator. Photo by Fred Sauceman.

procedures—blood tests, chest x-rays, a TB skin test, and an EKG.
That day from me alone, staff at Vanderbilt drew fifteen vials of
blood.

Based on all the information I was given at Vanderbilt, I felt
it unlikely that I would ever receive a deceased person's kidney.
My blood type is O. A person with that blood type can donate to
anyone but can only receive an O kidney. Therefore, those donors
with O blood, I learned, are in greatest demand.

That day I also met with a social worker for a psycho-social
evaluation. I had to sign a form stating that I had the financial
resources to cover the transplant and that I had a primary and a
secondary caregiver lined up, should I qualify for the transplant.

At the end of that eventful day, I met with nephrologist Dr.
Anthony Langone. I was concerned about having lupus and
whether it might disqualify me as a candidate for transplantation. He put those fears to rest by saying, "That's not even a factor

because the medication you would be taking after the transplant also helps keep lupus under control."

Every Monday morning at Vanderbilt, a team of doctors, nurses, transplant coordinators, and other health-care personnel reviews all the patients who are being evaluated for a possible kidney. "I tell patients all the time when I see them for evaluation that this is to determine if transplant is the right option for them," says Dr. Beatrice Concepcion, who would become my nephrologist. "When you're facing kidney disease, there are different options— conservative therapy, which is supportive care, versus dialysis, and what kind, or whether to pursue transplant. It depends on how sick the patient is, or how old, for example. Transplant may not be the best option. It can be a very rough course, and for someone who has severe heart disease and diabetes and peripheral vascular disease, that person may not necessarily do very well with a transplant. That's what we try to figure out by doing the evaluation and having the committee review everything."

Sometimes those Monday morning meetings involve the cases of as many as twenty patients. "There are black, white, and gray situations, which is why we have the committee," explains post-transplant coordinator Kristin Smith. "Significant and extensive cardiac disease, too much disease in vessels, and cancer are among the abnormal conditions that could result in a person being turned down. There is a social aspect as well. You have to have good support—somebody who's going to be there for all the doctors' visits, to be there while the patient is in the hospital, and to help with medications. And the patient has to be able to get here, to come to appointments. Many of our patients come from a good distance away."

As transplant coordinator Ashley Wilson puts it, "There are people who can't fill a gas tank to get here."

"Not just anybody can have a transplant," Kristin adds. "It's an amazing gift. You have to show that you want to be part of the process and are committed to it."

Ashley Wilson told us there are three possible outcomes from those Monday morning meetings. One is "appropriate," meaning that the person is a good candidate for a transplant. One is "decline." And the other is "deferred."

The first kidney transplant at Vanderbilt took place in 1962. The total number of kidney transplants since then is nearing 6,000. For the fiscal year ending June 30, 2016, Vanderbilt performed 239 kidney or kidney/pancreas transplants, 153 liver, 82 heart, and 26 lung. That represents an 18.5 percent increase over the previous year.

Among the additional requirements I had to meet before being evaluated by the transplant team were having a Pap test, mammogram, colonoscopy, and dental clearance. Fortunately, I was current on all those. I received a letter from Vanderbilt on November 23, 2013, instructing me to have a treadmill stress test at Johnson City Medical Center. I passed the test, and the results were sent to Vanderbilt. The transplant team reviewed those results and decided that even though my heart rate reached the maximum level, I reached that level in too short a period of time. That was not surprising to me because of my low activity level and the limitations of hip replacements that had lasted far beyond their predicted life span. My transplant coordinator called to tell me that the transplant team was concerned about my having lupus and that I needed further testing—more lupus blood work and a chemical stress test. All these came back normal.

The transplant team met again, and I received a call on December 11 from my transplant coordinator, who told me I had been approved for the transplant list. In a letter dated December 16, 2013, Paula Kilgore, transplant case manager with the insurance company Blue Cross Blue Shield of Tennessee, wrote, "We recently received a request from Dr. Anthony Langone to authorize your kidney transplant. Based on the facts your doctor gave us, this treatment is approved by your health benefit plan as of December 16, 2013, unless your condition changes." Two days later, Vanderbilt confirmed by letter that I had been placed on the active wait-list for a kidney transplant.

With the joy of that news came some additional information about my case. During the phone call, the transplant coordinator told me that because of all the blood transfusions I had had in my life, testing showed that I had developed a level of 78 percent antibodies in my blood that could attack a new kidney even of the same blood type. I later learned about an antibody desensitization treatment using a medication called IVIG—intravenous immunoglobulin. Its purpose is to reduce the transplant recipient's antibodies so that the new organ will be accepted. As nurse practitioner April DeMers puts it, "The IVIG is to wash your cells, to pull out any antibodies that might particularly react with your donor." I found that not every transplant center in the country uses IVIG. Vanderbilt does.

I began to learn all I could about how kidneys are matched and allocated nationwide. According to Vanderbilt University Medical Center's "Pre-Transplant Information Guide for Kidney and Pancreas Transplantation":

> If you do not have a living donor, you are placed on the national UNOS (United Network for Organ Sharing) wait-list. This is a list of people who are waiting for a deceased donor kidney. When you are listed on the registry, your name, tissue typing information (your antigens) and blood type (A, B, AB, or O) are placed in a computer. When a kidney becomes available, the computer prints a list of patients based on how long they have been waiting and the match between donor and recipient. It is unusual that two people would equally match the same kidney, but if this happens, and other considerations are also equal, the one who has been waiting the longest would get the kidney.

Being on the UNOS wait-list is essential for anyone searching for a kidney, whether from a living or deceased donor. Factors governing how soon patients can receive kidneys include how common their blood types and antigens are, the availability of kidneys, the presence of antibodies in the blood, and how long those patients have been on the wait-list. There are three primary tests to determine if patients and potential donors match: common blood typing, tissue typing, and cross-matching.

The transplant coordinator told me that because of my high level of antibodies, it could be anywhere from ten to fifteen years before I found a suitable match. She said, therefore, that my best bet would be to begin searching for a live donor. I felt that although I had gotten on the UNOS wait-list, there was really no way that I would ever be able to receive a deceased person's kidney. It was mandatory for me to begin the search for a live donor. And soon. My goal was to have a kidney transplant before I had to go on dialysis, and I knew time was running short. Recuperation times after kidney transplants are much shorter if the body has not undergone the stresses of dialysis. My glomerular filtration rate at the time I qualified for the wait-list was 13.

I think it's important to point out that making the wait-list is no guarantee that you will remain on it. Developing certain illnesses or diseases can potentially remove you from it. There are several requirements I had to follow once I got on the list. I was to notify my transplant coordinator of any illnesses or fevers or hospitalizations. Every month Vanderbilt sent me a kit with tubes and vials in it so that I could have a fresh supply of my blood drawn. That was necessary because antibodies can change from month to month, and the best blood sample possible was needed for typing and cross-matching with a potential donor. If a potential donor wanted to be tested, Vanderbilt would send a kit to me and the donor so that those kits could be returned simultaneously. The identity of any potential donors was not revealed to me by Vanderbilt. I only knew their identities if the potential donors themselves informed me of what they had done. My transplant coordinator only dealt with deceased persons' kidneys. A live-donor coordinator would contact me if my blood was needed to check for a match with a potential live donor. I was required to carry a cell phone with me constantly.

I began to consider how I was going to go about asking people to give me a kidney—those I knew and those I did not know. In my case, Vanderbilt's qualifications for a live donor were to have type O blood, to be less than 70 years old, to be without high blood pressure, to be without diabetes, and to be in good physical condition, with no other diseases or illnesses.

Facebook proved invaluable to us as a way to spread the word about my need for a kidney. This is my post from December 11, 2013:

> After almost 40 years of battling kidney disease caused by Systemic Lupus Erythematosus, I am now in kidney failure and have qualified for the kidney transplant program at Vanderbilt University Medical Center in Nashville, Tennessee. I am not on dialysis yet, but I'm about three percentage points away. Optimally, it would be best to get a kidney before my body becomes stressed from the dialysis process. Unfortunately, with my O type blood, I am told the waiting list for a deceased person's kidney is at least five to ten years. Therefore, a live donor would be the best chance for a kidney before I would have to be on dialysis. For these reasons, I am asking for your help. I need a kidney. If you have O blood, do not have high blood pressure, even if controlled by medication, do not have diabetes, and you are under 70 years old, would you consider being tested to see if you are a match for me? If so, you may contact Vanderbilt and tell them you want to be tested for Jill Sauceman. You can go to the website, www.vanderbilttransplantcenter.com, and click on the tab for Kidney Transplant Program, or you can call toll-free, 1-866-748-1491, and select option two. All information is confidential. If you should happen to be a match, your kidney is taken laparoscopically with a two-to-three-day hospital stay. My insurance will pay for this surgery. I have been able to lead a full life up until now. Stage 5 Chronic Kidney Disease makes me very

tired, and I have to pace myself and get plenty of rest. Fortunately, I have not experienced much swelling or nausea. I would like to have this surgery while I'm still in pretty good shape. I appreciate your consideration of this life-saving endeavor. May the Lord guide you as you make this decision.

More than seventy people shared that original post. After receiving so many responses, the next day I posted:

I am overwhelmed at the number of people and friends who wish they could qualify to be tested to donate a kidney for me. Just knowing you want to do it is a blessing. Thank you all for your prayers and for sharing my story. I feel confident that one day, I will get a call telling me that a match has been found. In the meantime, I ask for your continued prayers for me and for Fred.

We made use of the extensive network of contacts Fred had developed through the years with the region's news media. John Molley, managing editor of the *Johnson City Press* newspaper, enthusiastically volunteered to carry an article about me. Written by Jennifer Sprouse, it appeared on the front page on Friday, December 13, 2013, literally hours after I learned that I had made the wait-list. That same article also ran in the *Kingsport Times-News* the following Monday. We posted a link to the article on Facebook, and it was shared multiple times.

On Sunday, December 15, I announced to the congregation of Jonesborough Presbyterian Church that I had begun my quest for a kidney. I had read countless stories about people who had secured donors through church connections. Reverend Allen Huff, pastor at Jonesborough Presbyterian, immediately sent a mass email to the members of the church. At the same time, both Fred and I continued to make use of our respective Facebook pages to get word out about my need for a kidney. We received several responses from people willing to go through the testing. Some of them were matches and some were not.

A local medical doctor whom I did not know attempted to give me a kidney and progressed through the testing only to be turned down later because of a minor heart issue. And there were potential donors who simply got cold feet. One person pulled out because her spouse opposed it. In another case, a person told me that her spouse was against her donating a kidney, but she was still willing to take the next step for further testing if her kidney was a viable antigen-antibody match. She was saved from having to make that difficult choice when the results of her blood tests came back and showed that her kidney was not ideal.

I've never been a person who likes to ask for help, much less beg for it. Having to do this was one of the most difficult things I've ever done, knowing I was asking someone to give up a part of themselves in order to help me live. There were those who readily volunteered, but since I knew I had to have a large pool of candidates due to my odds, it was up to me to make such pleas to the general public. People from my part of the world, the Appalachian Mountains, generally don't like to be beholden to someone. Making this kind of request for help really ran against my inner nature, but circumstances demanded it. Most of the people who stepped up first did not have my blood type. Fred does not have my blood type.

We have made many friends over the years through our work in studying and writing about the foodways of Appalachia and the American South. Those treasured colleagues stepped up in a big way in our quest for a kidney. One of our most passionate advocates was friend and food writer Ronni Lundy, who wrote in February of 2014:

> Dear friends—My sweet friend Jill Derting Sauceman is battling lupus. She has been a fierce, joyful survivor for nearly four decades, but things have gotten severely worse in recent months. The short of it is, she needs a transplant, and she needs it quickly. She's on the waiting

list at Vanderbilt University in Nashville. You don't have
to live in Nashville to do this [be tested], but you would
have to travel there for the procedure. When I posted this
originally [the *Johnson City Press* article], some of you,
complete strangers to Jill, but complete angels, went in,
were tested, and didn't fully qualify. Love and gratitude
to you. It's possible that many folks who would care and
be able to do this didn't see it the first time, and things
are indeed getting more serious for Jill as time passes.
So search your hearts, search your kidneys. If you find
this is something speaking to you, respond. I would if I
could, but my health history precludes me. Jill and her
wonderful husband and my good friend and colleague
Fred Sauceman thank you for any help you can offer and
prayers and energy you can send their way. Thank you
all—Ronni.

January of 2014 was a quiet, uneventful month. My GFR
dropped to 12, but it rose to 13 the next month. Dr. Wiegand, my
Johnson City nephrologist, continued to stress the urgency of
potential donors getting to Vanderbilt to be tested as we fought
to keep me off dialysis. We knew that even if a match were found,
it could possibly take several months before the surgery would be
done.

With my suppressed immune system, I chose to spend January
and February hibernating at home in order to avoid getting the flu
and other viruses. I hadn't taken the flu shot because it had stirred
up my lupus several years before. We had a rough winter that year,
which made staying inside a little easier. I knew of at least three
people at the time who had been tested as possible donors, but
I was still in limbo. I tried to go on with my life's normal activities and even took the lead in planning my fortieth high school
reunion, which would take place in August of that year.

When I got that surprising telephone call from a Vanderbilt
kidney transplant coordinator at 6:30 one evening in late February of 2014, I was totally unprepared for the conversation that

followed. The coordinator asked me if I was at home, if I had been sick during the last forty-eight hours, and if I had transportation to be able to get to Nashville by midnight that night. I was at home, I had not been sick, and I had transportation. But I was totally taken aback by what she said next. "I wanted to let you know that we have a potential kidney available for you," she told me. Knowing that I had been cautioned to expect a ten-year wait and to rely on finding a live donor, I never even entertained the thought that a deceased person's kidney could become available so soon. Fewer than three months had passed since I was approved for the transplant wait-list.

Everything that I had been told and everything that I had read led me to believe that getting a live-donor kidney was more advantageous than getting a deceased-person's kidney. When the coordinator asked me if I would like to accept the kidney, if there were no complications, I did not know how to respond. I had not gotten to the point of desperation, and I knew I had potential live donors being tested. I asked the coordinator if it would be better to wait for a live-donor kidney. She then asked me the age of the most promising potential donor. When I told her the person was around 55 years old, she indicated that the deceased donor was in her thirties and that a kidney of that age was better than one more than half a century old.

The coordinator also told me that with this deceased donor, I would not have to have the IVIG treatment since the kidney was a perfect match. Since my brain was going in infinite directions and I could not give a definitive answer, the coordinator suggested that I go ahead and get my things together. She said the kidney would be biopsied that night. "You just prepare to head out the door, and we'll call you back and let you know whether it's a go or not," she said. "Then you can let us know your decision."

Shortly after the call, Fred arrived home from work. After I had time to think about it and Fred and I discussed it, I decided that I would accept the kidney. Not much time passed at all before the transplant coordinator called back and said the kidney had been biopsied. The tissue was sent to the lab, and a report came back that it checked out fine. I told her I was prepared to accept the kidney. As I was packing and we were about to head out the door, a third call came from Nashville. The transplant coordinator said the renal surgeon had examined the kidney and noted that it had been damaged. He did not think it was viable for a transplant. That was the deceased person's left kidney. The right kidney had already been designated for another woman, and medical personnel were waiting to do a cross-match, which is the last test done before transplant. The coordinator said if the cross-match was positive, the kidney could not be used for this woman and that I would be next in line for it. "If you hear back from me within the next thirty minutes, you'll know that the cross-match was positive, and if you don't, you'll know that it was negative and the other woman will receive the kidney," the coordinator said. I never heard back.

I may have felt slight disappointment, but, really, I had an overwhelming feeling of relief, for I still felt that a live-donor kidney would be the better option for me. I continued my quest to find one.

11

THE MAN WITH THE BRILLIANT BLOOD

—— FRED ——

"Who is Tina Elizabeth? Is that some showgirl you picked up somewhere?" Jill and I were on our way to eat steak dinners at The Butcher's Block, a popular restaurant in Greeneville, when she asked me those questions, prompted by an instant message she noticed on my iPhone. And then Jill saw, in that message, a reference to "your wife," which really caught her attention.

I quickly took the phone away from her to see what Tina had said. She wasn't a showgirl at all. She was a Facebook "friend" of mine, but one I barely knew. She had come forth with an incredibly generous offer of help. In that message, she asked me if it would be all right for her to communicate with Jill about helping to find her a live donor. I turned my phone over to Jill, and she and Tina "messaged" back and forth throughout our entire dinner. Tina volunteered to create a Facebook page for the sole purpose of seeking out a kidney. By the time we got back to Johnson City that night, the page was up and running. Tina Elizabeth Graham, who also has lupus, chose to call it "Jill's Journey: Quest for a Kidney." It was the first day of spring.

"I just felt driven to do that for you, especially after seeing Fred's post about what you were going through," Tina told Jill later. "I think God intended for me to see that. I didn't pay attention to all of his posts since I didn't know him personally, only because of the food stuff that he's known for and for his books. Somebody shared one of his posts a long time ago. And I thought, 'Wow, this man

writes books and knows about food and he lives in Johnson City!'
So I asked him to be a friend. When I saw his post about you, I just
think I was meant to see it that night. Nothing else mattered at that
point. You were all I could think about. I thought about myself and
thought about the fact that this could be me. The generosity in the
first few days of getting the page started was overwhelming. When
I contacted Fred, I was so afraid I would offend you. I didn't know
what kind of person you were. I was so conflicted. But now you
have helped me so much in my own battle with lupus."

—— JILL ——

In March of 2014, things had slowed down in my search, with
so many people being disqualified. The Facebook page was a huge
boost to our morale. By communicating just through instant mes-
saging, Tina showed me how to administer the page. I was aston-
ished that a total stranger would go to these lengths on my behalf.

With the coming of spring and the risk of flu lessening, I began
to get out more. I returned to church, where I resumed playing
handbells and singing in the choir. I had missed these activities
dearly.

My glomerular filtration rate was back down to 12. My hope
was that it would stay above 10 long enough to allow me to receive
a kidney before I was forced to start dialysis. I realized, though,
that it could take months, even with an available kidney, before
transplantation could occur. I was still very tired and wanted to
sleep a lot. Around this time, I started to experience a little nausea
but tried to remain upbeat.

In order to eliminate or at least reduce the nausea, I started
researching foods that should be eaten and foods that should be
avoided by someone experiencing kidney failure. I discovered that
foods to avoid include those high in potassium, phosphorus, and
protein. Consequently, I was relegated to what might be described
as "rabbit food." I continued to lose weight, but the new diet did
help with the nausea.

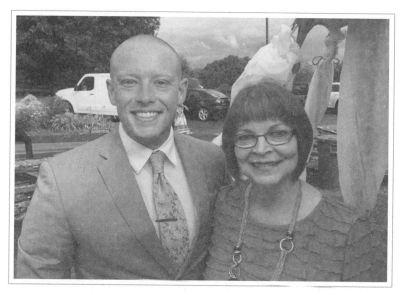

Jill's first face-to-face meeting with "honorary donor" Myles Cook in the summer of 2015. Photo by Fred Sauceman.

I drank a lot of hot lemon tea. My blood was bordering on acidosis, but I couldn't take sodium bicarbonate pills due to the nausea they caused. I searched for something to make my blood more alkaline. As strange as it sounds, lemons, even though acidic, turn alkaline when processed in the body. My breakfast, then, consisted of hot lemon tea and lemon biscotti. I only ate meat, in the form of a piece of chicken the size of the palm of my hand, about three times a week. It was clear, based on my discussions with Dr. Wiegand, that symptoms were going to drive the decision about dialysis, and I wanted to keep them to a minimum.

In preparing for the day when a kidney might become available, we had begun to think about what might happen on the home front in Johnson City, since there were people and animals who depended on us. One of those animals was a five-pound dog we named Lucy. In June of 1996, while looking for a dog for Fred's mother, we had rescued her from a questionable "kennel" in

Hawkins County, Tennessee. When that little one-pound puppy saw us that first day, she ran to Fred like a bullet out of a gun, seeming to say, "Get me out of here!" We did. She led a wonderful life with us, and on May 7, 2014, she turned 18 years old. She had become deaf and blind and infirm, but she was able to make that milestone. On June 9, 2014, with her veterinarian, Dr. James Robinson, we decided that Lucy had fulfilled her earthly mission, and we buried her in the backyard at our home.

Later that month, we made a return trip to one of our favorite places, New York City. I was concerned about my mobility, but by sleeping late and turning in early, we were able to have a fulfilling vacation. When we got back home, Fred received a message from Tina, asking if he could stop by her husband Donnie's place of employment and pick up something that she had for me. She had sent me an Origami Owl locket on a chain. The locket has four charms inside that are symbolic of four important facets of my life. Included with the locket was this note:

> Jill—Please wear this locket and keep your faith that a kidney will be found for you. The green ribbon is to bring awareness to your kidney disease and the purple ribbon to remind you of your long struggle with lupus. The faith charm will remind you that God is watching over you through all the struggles you have faced and will be facing. Finally, there is an angel wing to remind you that you are being watched over and prayed for by many angels out there. Wishing you well, my new friend. Hugs—Tina.

I received this wonderful gift just in time to wear it for my first television interview about my struggle to find a live kidney donor, with reporter Olivia Caridi of WCYB-TV, the NBC affiliate in Bristol, Virginia. I was able to show the locket and explain its significance in the news story that aired July 2. I was thrilled with this new gift and my new friend. We made a new friend in Olivia, too. She would eventually leave WCYB to be on ABC television's "The

Bachelor" and later would start a modeling and media career in New York. We met her for lunch at the Hourglass Tavern on West 46th Street in Manhattan almost two years after she interviewed me, and we asked her why my story had appealed to her so much.

"You were going to choir practice that evening," Olivia accurately remembered. "In typical reporter fashion, I said, 'Please, please, I'll meet you anywhere.' We met at a park, and you told me your story, which was really touching. I try to connect with people I'm interviewing, and so, of course, I wanted to stay in touch, and I followed your journey on Facebook. I remember meeting you for the first time. You had the sweetest smile and were such a sweet person, but I could tell you were malnourished and exhausted. I'd never seen energy like that in someone I knew was in pain. Your eyes were tired, and you were moving slowly. I sent a photo of you to my dad, who is a plastic surgeon. 'How does she look?' I asked him. 'She really needs a kidney,' he responded."

The WCYB-TV interview resulted in many more inquiries and people saying they were willing to be tested. Three of those inquiries ended up being good matches. Fred had shared the WCYB story on Facebook, and through one of his friends, a 27-year-old man named Myles Cook, in Elizabethton, Tennessee, saw the story. On July 3, he sent me a private message: "Jill, I will try calling [Vanderbilt] tomorrow morning and getting ahold of someone. If they are closed for the holiday, then I will try Monday morning. Are you aware of the testing/match procedure? It seems I could be a match. Do they test my blood (preliminarily) here or at Vanderbilt?"

I answered his questions and thanked him profusely. On July 11, I received another message from him: "Hey Jill, I received a packet of info today on donation from the Vanderbilt transplant department. Do you know when they generally send the blood test kit for me to take to the hospital? I'll call them Monday but thought you may know. Hope you are well."

The next day, I received another message from Myles: "Thanks for the info, Jill. I actually filled out the form online, and they contacted me via phone. They gave me all the directions for the blood kit and stated it was being sent. They stated it needed to be sent to them with the blood Monday through Wednesday."

On July 14, he said: "Called Vandy this morning and the blood kit is on its way. They stated they always send the info packet out immediately but that the blood test kit is mailed from a third party. I am really hoping and still praying." Later on that same day he told me that he was O+, young, and had a fairly low BMI (body mass index).

On July 25, Myles communicated with me again: "Hey Jill, I received the workup kit this evening. I'm leaving for vacation to South Carolina tomorrow, but to avoid waiting any longer, I am going to try and have it drawn and sent Monday from a local hospital in the area." I told Myles not to go to that trouble and that it would be fine if he waited until he was back home.

Then on August 4: "Hey Jill, I wanted to let you know the blood has been drawn and was sent off today from the UPS store." On August 12: "Hey, Jill. Vanderbilt called today. They stated I was a match, but that there was another possible donor who is further in the process than I. They stated they would call me back for further testing if that donor didn't work out for some reason."

The fortieth reunion of my Gate City High School class, which I had worked so hard to plan, took place on August 9 in Kingsport. I worked the entire day and night but made it through, serving as a smiling hostess despite being dragged down by my body. As it so happened, Fred's fortieth Greeneville High School reunion took place the very next weekend. (We are the same age, although I am three months and thirteen days older—a fact Fred occasionally brings up.)

On August 19, one of the live-donor coordinators called me from Vanderbilt and told me that the other possible donor, a female who had progressed farther through the testing process than Myles had, was applying for financial assistance to pay for her transportation, lodging, and meals to cover the time when she would go to Nashville for her physical workup. These preliminary travel expenses were not eligible for coverage through my insurance. Since I, as a potential recipient, didn't qualify for financial assistance myself, I was asked if I would volunteer to pay the preliminary travel expenses of this anonymous donor. I willingly agreed to do so. The coordinator indicated that she would tell the donor, and if that potential donor agreed to let us pay for those expenses, the coordinator would call me back. I heard nothing.

I managed to navigate the emotions and the arrangements surrounding Fred's mother's death on August 23. Her graveside service was held on a beautiful late summer day in the cemetery where generations of Fred's mother's family are buried.

Around the first of October, WCYB-TV contacted me again, wishing to do a follow-up story. I asked Vanderbilt about the anonymous donor since six weeks had passed with no word. Another live-donor coordinator told me that the lady in question who was to come for a physical workup was "timid" about my paying for her transportation to Vanderbilt. Apparently, for whatever reason, this potential donor, who had gotten so far into the process, decided to abandon her effort.

This was undoubtedly the most frustrating period throughout my entire search for a kidney. Things didn't seem to be moving at all. I fully realized I wasn't the only person waiting for a kidney, but I knew that I had three potential donors who were good matches and the second in line had not been contacted. On the advice of Vanderbilt, I asked Myles to get in touch with a live-donor coordinator to determine his status, and he did.

On the morning of October 8, I got a call from a live-donor coordinator telling me she was sending blood kits for both Myles and me, to be returned on October 20. We both had blood drawn, shipped it off that day, and informed each other that we had done so.

That remarkable fall, death, somehow, made way for life. We continue to be amazed by how things fell into place for us during that year of 2014, although three of those events caused us great pain. Lucy died in June, Fred's mother died in August, and in October, we lost our cat. "Our cat," though, is a bit misleading. For years, a tortoise-shell feline named Chloe had walked across

Osceola Street to snag treats in our driveway. She belonged to the Grogg family. When the Groggs welcomed more cats, Chloe elected to cross that street again, permanently, to avoid the competition. We kept her for about two years before she had to leave this world on October 20.

On the evening of October 24, Fred and I were driving from Kingsport to Johnson City on Highway 36 after stopping at an Ingle's store, in search of some Terra Yukon Gold potato chips, when a message came through my iPhone. It was Myles.

"Got some great news today!" That was all he said, leaving me in suspense. I asked him if he could share that news. "Yes," he answered. "They said my blood was 'brilliant.' They used a lot of technical language I'm not familiar with, but they said it should work with your antibodies. They will be calling me to set up the day of testing in Nashville. Looks like I will have to quit working out for a while and change the diet up a bit, though, to lower proteins in the blood. I'm excited. Looking forward to it."

Four days later, Myles let me know that Vanderbilt had called and had scheduled the earliest possible date for testing, which was December 9.

I thought, "How many 27-year-old people would do this—would give up a part of their body to help me survive?" I felt both gratitude and guilt. How could I ask such a young man, who wasn't even married yet, to have this surgery? When I found out what he did for a living, it began to make more sense to me. He worked for the Carter County Sheriff's Office in Northeast Tennessee. Putting other peoples' lives ahead of their own is just standard practice for law-enforcement people. "Thank you," multiplied exponentially, just didn't seem to be enough. Myles kept me informed, kept me looking up, and never expressed a bit of doubt as we headed toward that important December 9 testing date.

As promising as his situation seemed, I never stopped trying to recruit donors. My next step was to get people interested in a program called paired donation. Here's how it works, as described in a communique from Vanderbilt:

In paired donation transplantation, two patient-and-donor pairs (A and B) that do not match are identified. The donor of pair A must be identified to be compatible with the recipient of pair B. Additionally, the donor of pair B must be identified to be compatible with the recipient of pair A. This allows each paired recipient to receive a kidney transplant. Through the Alliance for Paired Donation, Vanderbilt Transplant Center has access to all of their potential donors and recipients in the United States. If you have any potential living donors or if you had living donors that tested for you previously and were told they were incompatible but are still interested in helping you receive a kidney through the Alliance for Paired Donation, please feel free to have them contact us.

In other words, if I have somebody to donate for me who is not compatible, and Jane Doe has somebody who wants to donate to her and that person is not compatible, our donors would be tested to see if they are compatible with each of us. Then, I would get her donor's kidney, and she would get my donor's kidney. We would both end up with kidneys, and our donors would still be able to donate.

12

"REPORT TO THE SEVENTH FLOOR CRITICAL CARE TOWER"

—— JILL ——

It's funny how you remember the most seemingly insignificant things that surround momentous events. As I was preparing for that church luncheon in Jonesborough on Sunday, November 9, I got a call from our home-security company indicating that we had a faulty motion sensor. I scheduled an appointment for the technicians to come to our house the following afternoon, November 10. While I was waiting for them to arrive, that 1:55 P.M. call came from Vanderbilt. I was sitting on the couch. It was Margot Chaffin, a transplant coordinator I had never talked to before. After I answered her questions, she said, "I am happy to be the one to call and tell you that we have a kidney available for you." We talked about the additional testing that had to be done, and she told me she would be calling back. She instructed me to begin collecting my belongings and to await that second call.

After I summarized the call for Fred, I called my sister Joyce Summers and gave her an assignment. I asked her to break the news to my mother who, I knew, would be overly emotional. Honestly, Fred and I didn't have time for much emotion that afternoon. Our mission was to keep calm and get down to the business of preparing to get on the road. We notified neighbors and asked them to get our mail and newspapers. I shared the news with our pastor, and I informed Dr. Wiegand's office, since he had been such an integral part of my care.

In order to get to Nashville by 9:00 Central (10:00 Eastern), I targeted 5:00 Eastern as our departure time. As I was packing and making calls, the technicians from the alarm company arrived! I gave them a quick explanation of the problem we were having and told them why I was trying to get out of town. When they had fixed the malfunction in the alarm system and were attempting to tell me what they had done to correct it, a second call came in from Margot Chaffin at Vanderbilt, at 3:30, as Fred was finishing up his newscasts. I texted him at WETS-FM to tell him about the call: "I've got wonderful news," Margot said. "The tissue match and the biopsy of the kidney turned out beautifully. It looks like it's a perfect match." Margot added that the kidney was from a very young person who had just died.

I could hardly believe that with my level of antibodies, a perfect-match kidney could be found in that short a period of time. I had been on the wait-list for less than a year. There was absolutely no hesitation on my part this time. Margot again asked if I could get to Nashville between 9:00 and 10:00 Central time, because, she said, the surgeon was contemplating performing the surgery that evening. She said it could either be that night or the next morning, but she wanted me there just in case.

"I know all your instructions say to report to the Emergency Room," Margot said. "But I want you to go straight to the Seventh Floor Critical Care Tower."

I hung up the phone, apologized to the alarm system technicians for their wait, and explained to them what I had just been told. Before we left home, I posted on the "Jill's Journey: Quest for a Kidney" Facebook page: "Vanderbilt called. They have a kidney that is a perfect match for me. It is from a very young person. Thank you for all your prayers." That post alone reached 6,488 people.

The first person to respond was Laurell Millirons from Dallas. She had undergone a kidney transplant with a live donor in 2013. I was introduced to her by a college friend from Greeneville,

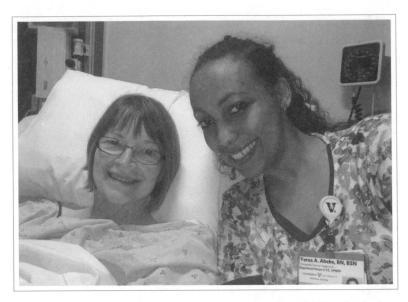

Jill right after her transplant, with Yerus Abebe, RN. Photo by Fred Sauceman.

Tennessee, Becky Benko Chamberlain. Through that Facebook page, Laurell was a constant source of advice and encouragement during my wait for a kidney. "Tell Fred to grab a notebook and pen from the gift shop," she said. "You guys will want to write down everything. It all becomes a blur, and you can forget things along the way. Write down good nurses' names, medications, gifts, calls, questions, and visitors. I'm here if you have questions."

I told her that Fred keeps a reporter's notebook with him at all times. We indeed did document countless details, enabling us to write this book.

After that Facebook post, the first person to send me a private message was Myles, who told me he was praying about my recent news and that he would wait to make sure everything worked out before he cancelled his physical on December 9.

"Hi everyone. Wanted to update you on Jill," wrote Tina Graham on my kidney page. "She is on her way to Nashville, to Vanderbilt. They're in Cookeville, Tennessee, now. She left Johnson

City around 5:00 P.M. Eastern time, so making good time. I asked her if she was nervous, and she said, 'No, just excited.'"

As we drove to Nashville that night, we talked about the events that had led up to the trip and how things had fallen into place for us so remarkably well. Our dog Lucy's death at age 18 the preceding June, Fred's mother's death in August at age 91, and our adopted cat Chloe's passing at age 18 in October somehow seemed to pave the way for this moment. We missed each of them terribly, but in all three cases, it was time. We felt like our lives had been guided and orchestrated toward a crescendo. We had even started a huge remodeling project at our home in the spring of 2014, adding a new sunroom and spa room and renovating our den and one of our bathrooms. Part of the renovation was the addition of a washer and dryer in that bathroom in October so that I would not have to climb stairs. At a time when we both needed father figures, a genial and talented contractor named Glen Whittington came into our lives to do the work. He was 79 years old at the time. He and his colleagues, Denny Dugger and Fred Jenkins, were in our home just about every day from April until November of 2014. They became a part of the family. We laughed with them and joked with them and absorbed their wisdom and guidance daily. And when they were all done, I had comfortable new quarters that would serve me well during my recuperation.

We made it to Vanderbilt University Medical Center by 9:00 Central time. One seemingly small detail that night came to define our entire experience at Vanderbilt. Fred hadn't been in the hospital there since his father's brain-tumor surgery in January of 1972. We had no idea where to park the car. When we arrived, we saw a "Valet Parking" sign right outside the hospital. An attendant greeted us, asked if we needed directions, and parked our car, without a fee. Attendants were even instructed not to take tips. The kindness and patient-centered focus we experienced that night continues to this day, no matter where we go in the hospital or clinic.

THE CRITICAL HOURS BEFORE TRANSPLANT

Dr. Douglas Hale, Transplant Surgeon:

By law, Medicare requires all hospitals to identify potential organ donors when somebody deteriorates and goes into brain death or has cardiopulmonary failure. Anyone who looks like they're heading in that direction, there's an obligation on the part of the hospital to notify the local OPO (Organ Procurement Organization).

The OPO is the organization that is chartered by UNOS (United Network of Organ Sharing) to secure the organs. And so then that OPO will send out a coordinator to evaluate the patient and determine if they are a suitable donor, and if they are a suitable donor, then the OPO notifies UNOS and obtains all the laboratory tests that are necessary for the allocation system. Once UNOS has that information, it runs the list, and that list will determine who the heart recipient is, the lung recipient, the liver, the kidneys, pancreas—for whatever organs are going to be procured and deemed usable, UNOS will then generate a nationwide list of the recipients.

Once UNOS generates that list, that's when we hear. So there's been a lot of work going on already before we even know that there's anything going on. And we'll get notified that we have an individual who is number two on the list or number four on the list. And the OPO will post the donor information on a website that we can access and we can look at all the different variables that go into determining whether or not the organ is suitable for use.

And then we'll make a decision, whether it's worthwhile pursuing. That's when the coordinators will typically call the patient and say, "Hi. How are you? Are you doing fine or have you been in the hospital? Have you been sick recently? Is everything okay? Because there's an organ out there and it's going to be possibly heading in your direction."

Then it typically will take another half a day or so before the smoke clears and all of the institutions that are being offered the organs—some of them will turn them down, some of them will accept them—and so it takes maybe about ten, twelve hours or so before the list matures and you know who's really going to be number one for the organ and who's going to be really number two. So you may start off at number twelve, but if the eleven people ahead of you can't get a transplant for a variety of reasons, you'll wind up being eventually number one.

And then usually about that time that everything is maturing, at the same time they're figuring out when the person is going to be going to the OR for the procurement. Typically what happens is the institution that is going to receive the liver sends the procuring surgeons, and so they will procure the liver, the kidneys, and the pancreas.

Once we know when the OR time is, we'll have a general idea of when the organ is going to get here, because we can just plot out distance. We figure out how far away the patient lives and how soon we'll have a cross-match. That's when we figure out when to have the patient come in so that they're here and ready to go by the time the organ gets here and we can go to the OR. That's the flow. And it happens many times a week.

When we checked into a temporary two-patient room that night, the first person we saw was a young registered nurse from Ethiopia, Yerus Abebe. I don't think a smile left her face the entire time she was with us. Bright and enthusiastic, she is in the right line of work. She had worked in a kidney dialysis unit after graduating from Selam Nursing College in Addis Ababa. She had been working at Vanderbilt for a year and called it her "dream job." She explained to us that transplants did not take place in Ethiopia—just dialysis, which, she said, was very expensive. Ethiopian patients, she told us, had to go to another country, such as Thailand, for transplantation, and they had to have live donors. Our conversation with Yerus increased our gratitude for the gift we were about to be given.

Yerus began the workup for the final testing before the transplant. At 10:35 P.M., nephrologist Dr. Rafia Chaudry came into the room and told us that the cross-match was negative, which is the result we wanted. The surgeon then had to check the anatomy of the kidney. Surgery was planned for the next morning, around 6:00 or 7:00. It couldn't come soon enough, for I learned that night that my GFR had dwindled down to a mere 8. A few more weeks or maybe even days, and I would have been on dialysis.

"Long night, I know," Laurell posted on my kidney page. "But it's nothing compared to the gift I trust you will receive this morning. We lost count of the miracles in my transplant process. I am sure you will, too."

Fred decided to stay in the room and sat up in a chair all night. I was able to sleep a little, but he was not, from a combination of anticipation and the fact that the patient on the other side of the curtain had a heavy finger on the television remote control and also spent the night telling stories. We learned in great detail about how he had been struck by lightning while he was working on a commode.

I was taken down to surgery at 6:20 A.M. on Veterans Day and first met my transplant surgeon, Dr. Douglas Hale, a United States Army veteran who had performed kidney transplants at Walter Reed National Military Medical Center in Bethesda, Maryland. Dr. Hale is the son of an automobile mechanic from Buffalo, New York, and a graduate of Georgetown University School of Medicine. Like me, he did not come from a privileged background. The Army made his medical education possible.

"Don't be surprised if you wake up on dialysis," Dr. Hale told me that morning. "Sometimes it takes twenty-four to forty-eight hours or even longer for the kidney to wake up." After going to such great lengths to avoid dialysis, I couldn't help thinking I would be disappointed if it did occur after the surgery.

—— FRED ——

After we spoke to the surgeon, I walked to the waiting room and checked the monitors every few minutes for updates. Thomas Williams, a person I had come to know through my work with the Southern Foodways Alliance, sat with me that morning. He was there when the message came across the monitor, well before 10:00, that Jill was successfully out of surgery. The operation had taken fewer than three hours.

"Great news indeed! I saw Fred Sauceman this morning at VUMC," Thomas posted on Facebook. "What a great couple and love story. Our continued prayers for Jill Derting Sauceman and her recovery. Hopefully before long, she will be making that dried apple stack cake that I'm so fond of again."

By lunchtime, Jill was eating chicken parmigiana and that new kidney was working perfectly. We were told that as soon as the ureter and blood vessels were hooked up, urine production started. Miraculously, there was no need whatsoever for the dreaded dialysis.

That afternoon, Jill met her new nephrologist, Dr. Beatrice Concepcion, a young, energetic doctor from the Philippines, and we bonded with her immediately. "You've done as well as you can hope for," she said, smiling. "You got a great donor kidney from a young person that matched you very well. And it worked immediately. You got something just as good as a living donor."

—— JILL ——

That day, too, my nurse, Jessica Walker, brought me what everyone commonly called the "kidney bible." I would refer to this publication of the Vanderbilt Transplant Center constantly over the ensuing months. It's a manual provided to all transplant recipients with rules and instructions on how to live your life in order to protect the new organ.

"You must take responsibility for your own care, both in the hospital and when you go home," the manual reads. "You need to be more aware of your body now more than ever before. There is a lot for you to learn. Nobody expects you to know it all at once. We do expect you to put your best effort to learn and be independent. Your doctors and nurses will help you along the way. However, the most important member of the team is YOU. Without your full cooperation and participation, the team's best efforts cannot succeed."

I was told that one of the major reasons for organ rejection was failure to adhere to the regimen of taking medications regularly. I vowed then and there never to deviate from that regimen.

Highlighted in yellow in that "kidney bible" are these rules:

• Follow your medication schedule.
• Keep all of your scheduled appointments, both for the doctor and for blood work.
• Develop healthy habits. This means eating healthy, getting regular exercise, and developing healthy ways to cope with stress.
• Communicate effectively with your family and the transplant team.

I've kept this manual close at hand for more than three years now. Included in it are things to watch for when you go home that might indicate rejection, such as a temperature higher than 100.5, nausea, vomiting, dark, tea-colored urine, sore throat, and excessive weight gain. There is a list of both prescription and over-the-counter medications that transplant patients should avoid, as well as dietary guidelines. And there is a chart for recording blood pressure and temperature twice a day, weight once a day, and urine output, which I measured for six weeks after returning home.

Dr. Hale came to my room after the surgery to tell me that the procedure had gone perfectly. My creatinine, which had risen to 5.27 before the transplant, was already coming down. At 9:37

A.M., right after surgery, it was 3.83 and my GFR 12. By 7:50 P.M.: creatinine 3.43, GFR 14.

I was under constant watch. For the first twenty-four hours after a transplant, the nurse to patient ratio is 1:1. "You're in there every hour," said Ashley Wilson, one of my nurses who is now a transplant coordinator. "It's not an ICU floor, but it's ICU-level care. The biggest thing is urine output, because that's something you have to monitor constantly. A lot of patients get deceased donor kidneys that don't automatically work. That can go on for hours to days and in some cases, to my understanding, it can go on for weeks at a time."

Later we asked nurse practitioner April DeMers about the risks and dangers to watch for after the transplant. "It's rare here, but you always run the risk of the graft not working," she said. "The biggest risk of causing organ failure is clots. If the new organ is cut off from the blood supply, it dies, and that can happen quickly, within twenty-four hours. Of course you always worry about bleeding. We don't see a lot of rejection in the first six to eight weeks because of the medicines we use, but you never really cannot worry about rejection. The highest risk is in the first ninety days. Certain populations are more likely to reject. The African American population requires a little bit more medication to suppress the immune system. We don't know why. Some Asian populations are the same. Finally, a lot of the rejection we see is in noncompliance—people just don't do what we tell them to."

Post-transplant coordinator Kristin Smith told me later: "It's a major surgery, but you seemed to do so well even the first day post-op—sitting up in bed, smiling. It's like you couldn't even tell that you'd had major surgery."

Dr. Hale gave me another bit of news. He said the deceased person from whom I had received the kidney was 27 years old. Myles Cook, my potential live donor, was the exact same age.

By 4:00 the morning after surgery, my numbers had continued to improve. The creatinine was down to 2.55, and my GFR had risen to 19, the highest it had been in years.

"We've seen firsthand, over the last two days, why Vander-bilt University Medical Center is among the best in the world," Fred wrote on Facebook. "Every base is covered, every contingency is prepared for. I am deeply impressed with everyone who has helped us through the transplant. Quick update on Jill: The surgeon was by this morning. He indicated that she is doing very well. The surgery itself only lasted about two hours. We got her up and walked her late last night. Today she undergoes a treatment by IV that is intended to negate an antigen in the donor's blood serum. This was no surprise, though. I was able to get some sleep last night and even found time this morning for a breakfast of lox, eggs, onions, and a bagel at Noshville."

Later that morning, Jill wrote: "I am now taking the IVIG treatment to keep me from rejecting the donated kidney. So far no problems. The only negative thing about this surgery is that they pump a lot of fluid into you while the surgery is going on. When I got on the scales this morning, my nurse told me not to be surprised by the weight gain. Sure enough, I had gained fifteen pounds. At least I have a good kidney to get rid of all this fluid."

The IVIG treatment lasted for five hours. The dosage was increased every hour. Nurses loaded me up on IV Benadryl, IV steroids, and Tylenol just before administering the treatment, which I tolerated well.

HOW IS TRANSPLANT SURGERY DONE

FRED: Take me through the major steps that are involved in transplanting a kidney.

DR. DOUGLAS HALE: The donor operation, typically for kidneys, is done locally, because the tendency is to allocate the kidneys local to where they are being procured to minimize the ischemia time. We are getting away from that a little bit because preservation is a little bit better, and they are trying to reduce the disparity in waiting times between different regions of the country.

What will happen is the kidneys are removed, they are flushed on the back table, and then, depending upon the age of the donor, they are also biopsied and they are looked at under a microscope. And so we will get a final piece of information that says this is what the anatomy of the kidneys is, this is how many veins, how many arteries, this is what they look like. And then we'll also get the biopsy results, and that's when we make the final acceptance of the organ. Then the Organ Procurement Organization (OPO), that up to this point was in charge of taking care of the donor, getting him or her to the OR, now is in charge of getting the kidney from one place to the other. So they will arrange transportation, either by commercial jet or courier, depending upon how far away it is, and we'll be told when the organ is going to arrive here. Knowing that information, we typically work to have the recipient here before the kidney is going to arrive, usually by several hours so that we can do all the testing and make sure that the recipient is ready to go. And then probably the easiest part of the whole process happens, and that's the surgery. We tell the operating room we'll have an organ and the recipient at this time, and this is the time we'd like to go. And we usually go within a few hours of that time. A kidney transplant takes about three hours. Maybe a couple of hours in the recovery room after that. Three days in the hospital and then out.

FRED: What are the technical challenges in this surgery as far as dexterity is concerned and those kinds of skills you have to develop as a surgeon?

DR. HALE: The most technically challenging aspects of transplant surgery have to do with the nature of the tissue you're working with. And so for an average, run-of-the-mill first-time transplant, where you're going into tissue that hasn't been manipulated before, and where there's good anatomy, it's a relatively straightforward and simple operation. We sew a vein together with a vein, an artery with an artery, and then the ureter directly to the bladder. These are all relatively standardized. We don't do it that much differently than the way it was done back in the 1950s. Where the real challenge comes in is when you are putting the transplant into somebody who's had three prior transplants and everything is scarred. Or somebody who has very limited blood vessel availability and there's a lot of calcium in the blood vessels. We try to mitigate the challenge by being very thorough in our evaluation beforehand so that we know, when we open up, that there's only a very short segment of vessel available for use—that we're opening up in such a way that that segment is available to us and we're not going in finding out that nothing's usable and we have to go over to the other side and look over there. The hardest thing is dealing with reoperative surgery.

FRED: How do you sew vein to vein, artery to artery? How is that done?

DR. HALE: It's called end-to-side technique. The kidney comes with a vein hanging off of it. We take the end of that vein, and you have a vein in your body that runs in the pelvis. We just control it with clamps above and below, and we make a little slit in the vein. Then we take the end of that other vein, put it down there, and sew them together. We use a standard vascular suture that's about the size of a hair. The connection itself is maybe a good inch, typically, of the vein. The artery is usually much smaller. That is about a third of an inch.

FRED: Is the kidney always placed in the front?

DR. HALE: We place it anywhere on either of the external iliacs, which is down in the pelvis, the common iliacs, which is a little higher in the pelvis, or especially in small children, we'll put it directly on the aorta and the vena cava, which is directly in the abdomen. For the vast majority of cases, it goes pretty deep in the pelvis, right next to the bladder. It makes it nice and easy to connect it. Your intestines are enclosed in a big sac, and so we go through your abdominal wall layers, and we just take that sac, the whole sac, and we push it up out of the way. We put the kidney in, and then the whole sac just kind of falls back on top of it.

FRED: You told me that your father was an automobile mechanic and that your hobby is working on cars. Are there any common connections between working on cars and working on bodies?

DR. HALE: One hundred percent. It is. I get the same satisfaction in sitting over an engine and systematically taking it apart and putting it back together that you get in the operating room. There is 100 percent crossover. My plan was to do heart surgery, and then at the beginning of my fourth year of training, I did six months of research, and during that six months of research, I did a bunch of transplants in monkeys. And that's what got me hooked—seeing organs gray, lifeless, cold, and plugging them in and watching them come back to life. There's nothing like it.

FRED: The day after Jill's transplant, she was given the IVIG treatment. Not every transplant center does that, right?

DR. HALE: Correct.

FRED: Explain how that works.

DR. HALE: There is a variety of different scenarios in which it is used. The basic goal of IVIG is to convince your body to stop making antibodies. And then the other aspect of what it's doing is something called binding of anti-idiotype antibodies. And so the only individuals who get IVIG are individuals who have preexisting antibodies that we think may attack the kidney. We want your body to stop making antibodies so we flood your body with a bunch. That shuts off your production. Your body sees that there's a surplus of antibodies floating around and it stops producing them.

FRED: When Jill checked into the hospital, her GFR was 8, but she had not been on dialysis. How unusual is that?

DR. HALE: Eight is pretty low. Normally folks are starting dialysis between 10 and 15. What drives starting dialysis is mostly symptoms, and if you were at 8 and you weren't having symptoms, you were just very lucky.

FRED: Jill's kidney damage was caused by lupus. How often do you see that?

DR. HALE: It's in the low single digits in terms of the overall percentage of cases. The vast majority of folks we see are hypertension, diabetes, primary glomerular disease, and so lupus would be down there. We probably do five to ten a year.

FRED: When you see a patient like her who has done so well as a result of the work of the team here at Vanderbilt, how does that make you feel?

DR. HALE: It makes us all feel good. What we're doing makes a difference. It's a great feeling to take care of folks and to have them do well. It's frustrating when they don't do well. And under those circumstances, our solace is we tried as hard as we could to get them a good outcome and just sometimes it's out of our hands. Thank goodness the good outcomes far outnumber the bad.

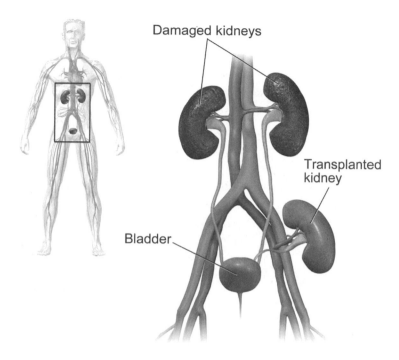

Kidney Transplant

Source: *BruceBlaus, Blausen Medical Communications; CC BY-SA 4.0, https://commons.
wikimedia.org/w/index.php?curid= 44925836*

—— FRED ——

More news from Room 7T3: "Jill is now unhooked from all telemetry and is walking frequently," I wrote. "Her creatinine, which had been hovering around 5 pre-transplant, is now at 1.5 and her GFR has climbed to 35."

—— JILL ——

"Day two post-op, still puffy from all the IV fluids they have been giving me, but the IVs are all out now," I wrote. "I feel great, except for a sore esophagus from being intubated during the surgery. The surgeon took my bandages off and removed the drainage tube. He said everything looks wonderful. I'm still planning to be discharged tomorrow but will stay in Nashville, close to Vanderbilt, until Monday, when I have my follow-up clinical visit. I should be home by Tuesday and will have to return every week for the next month for checkups and adjustments to medication. Nurses will be coming in to discuss diet and medication. The transplant team continues to be amazed that I have never been on dialysis. I have had the best nurses and doctors. I will be doing everything they say in order to keep this precious gift that came from another family's loved one."

Nurse practitioner April DeMers and post-transplant coordinator Kristin Smith came to visit me that afternoon, reviewing again the contents of the "kidney bible" and what my discharge orders would be. "Nobody would ever know you've battled what you have," April told me later. "You don't look like you've had anything done. I think if I passed you in the supermarket, I'd never know that you'd ever been sick a day in your life."

I found out that Kristin not only had the medical training to help patients through transplantation, she also had very close personal experience. Her mother had a transplant three years earlier, with the help of a live donor, Kristin's sister's best friend. Like me, she received her kidney just shortly before she would have gone on dialysis.

April would provide continuity of care for me as I transitioned from hospital to home. "My first physical contact with the patient is the day of the transplant or the day after, when people are awake and able to talk," she said. "I carry them from that point to about six weeks post-op. And then if people have wound issues or surgical complications, I follow them until those are resolved."

I began to learn more about what I should and should not eat. Number one on the banned list is grapefruit. There is a naturally occurring chemical in both grapefruit and blood orange that interferes with the absorption of the transplant medications, and does the same with statins and other medications. Jane Greene, a Vanderbilt dietitian who works solely with kidney patients, says that so many medications are affected by grapefruit that the hospital's food service department made the decision to eliminate it entirely from all menus—no juice, no segments, no grapefruit halves coming out at breakfast.

Because of my compromised immune system, any beef that I am to be served has to be at least cooked to medium well. Eggs should be solid, not runny. I was told not to eat at any buffets or salad bars because of the risk of bacteria when so many people handle and pass over the food. I was told to wash every fruit and vegetable, and I was instructed to avoid dairy products that had not been pasteurized. I was given a list of foods high in magnesium, potassium, and phosphorus, since the transplant medications tend to deplete them. One doctor told me, "I want you to go back to your hotel room and order a pizza and eat it along with a big Coke," because I needed the phosphorus from the carbonated beverage and a little calcium from the cheese. I hadn't consumed a Coke since 2008. One of the most important things that the hospital staff constantly mentioned was to drink two to three liters of water per day. The kidneys should always be flushed out so bacteria are not allowed to grow, causing a kidney or bladder infection. Such an infection could be potentially harmful to the kidney and lead to rejection.

"There are some dietitians who don't want anything to do with renal patients because it is so complicated in trying to figure out what they can eat," Jane Greene said. "From a nutritional standpoint, the kidneys are a challenge."

I chose not to dwell on the very minor restrictions but to think about all the foods I could eat that I had been forced to avoid for so long. Transplant patients are normally placed on a sodium-restricted diet, but because this young kidney I received was doing such a great job of carrying sodium out of my body, my blood pressure was tending to drop too low—this in a person whose blood pressure once topped out at 234/132. In a radical departure from the past, I was told not to worry about sodium.

My room was a busy place that Thursday, November 13. A team from the Vanderbilt Pharmacy came to discuss all my medications with me. The two antirejection medications are Prograf and Myfortic. These are medicines that I will take for the entire life of the kidney. The Myfortic dosage never changes, but Prograf levels are adjusted downward over a period of months. For antirejection as well as anti-inflammation, I began taking 20 milligrams of prednisone, eventually tapering off to five, the dosage that I will remain on. For a few months, I took Dapsone, which prevents bacterial infections. For six months, I took Valcyte, a drug that is intended to prevent viral infections. Pharmacists also recommended that I take a medicine to prevent acid reflux, because of all the medications I was on. That is usually Prilosec, but I was already taking Nexium because of a prior esophageal ulcer in 2008 and just stayed on that.

Among my other temporary restrictions, I could not lift any more than five pounds for two months in order to protect the surgical site.

My doctors and nurse practitioners cautioned me to stay away from crowds for several months because I would be highly susceptible to viruses as a result of the antirejection medications. I was told that anyone with a cough or the sniffles should not visit me, and anyone touching me must first use hand sanitizer—not forever, but just during the critical period for rejection. Knowing that I should not risk being sick as I was seeking a kidney, in October of 2014 I received my first flu shot since 1980. Having an up-to-date flu vaccine is a requirement before anyone can be considered for an organ transplant.

—— FRED ——

By the time of Jill's transplant, reports were already coming in that flu cases could hit epidemic proportions during the 2014/2015 flu season. The flu season had started early that year, with the predominant flu strain being H3N2. That year's flu vaccine would turn out to be less effective than usual because the virus mutated after the shot was developed and manufactured. The National Institute of Allergy and Infectious Diseases reported that it was only 33 percent effective in preventing the flu. I'm sure we went through a few gallons of hand sanitizer that winter. By late December, the number of flu deaths in the United States did indeed reach epidemic levels, according to the Centers for Disease Control and Prevention.

13

DISCHARGE DAY

—— JILL ——

November 14, 2014, after breakfast: "Day three post-op. I am being discharged today. The catheter is out, and my new kidney is working perfectly. They have given me some Lasix to quickly get me back to the weight I was before all the IV fluids. So I'll be getting up frequently going to the bathroom. My goal is to be out of here by early afternoon. I have a follow-up visit on Monday, so we are staying in Nashville until Tuesday."

Dr. Concepcion came by my room and said everything looked great. My creatinine was down to 0.9, the lowest in ten years. The GFR was 60, the highest in ten years. All the electrolytes were perfect as well.

"We will be returning to Nashville on Mondays or Tuesdays for clinical checkups for the next six weeks," I noted. "Then the visits will be reduced to every other week, every three weeks, every month, every two months, and so on. If all goes well, I will eventually come to Vanderbilt only once a year."

"I can't say enough about the excellent care I have received from the whole kidney transplant team," I wrote to my Facebook friends on discharge day. "It's a top-notch program. They are all amazed at how well I've done so quickly. God bless you all for your prayers, thoughts, calls, and uplifting comments. You don't know how much it helps me to get through this whole process. The nurses can't believe how little pain medication I took. I just left it up to the Good Lord to see me through, and He was by my side all the way. I'll be looking forward to the day when I can be out and about, reconnecting with all my friends and loved ones. In the meantime, there is always social media. Thank you all and God bless."

Perhaps my joy over the success of the operation masked my pain, but the amount of soreness I felt was bearable. I don't recall taking any pain medication past the next morning after surgery. I was given prescriptions for pain medications to take home, but I did not use them.

Before lunch I took a shower, unassisted, and washed my hair. I packed my things, allowed that new kidney to perform several times, and awaited discharge. I was given a bright green bag with "Donate Life" printed on it. Like the kidney bible, this bag is still rarely out of my sight. It contained a plastic medication tray for measuring out pills and capsules a week at a time, a blood pressure machine, thermometer, and what the nurses called "the urine hat," to keep track of kidney output.

Discharge papers arrived, and transport came to wheel me down to the main hospital lobby, where we waited on one of those much-appreciated valets to retrieve our car. On the second day in Nashville, Fred had managed to secure a room at the Hilton Garden Inn not far from the Vanderbilt campus. With the amazing growth of Nashville, oftentimes booking a room is a challenge, but after several calls, he had found a comfortable one. He told me he learned to say "kidney transplant" in Spanish so that he could let the hotel staff know I needed special care. I walked the halls of the hotel in order to build my strength and slept well that night with no interruptions.

"It's bittersweet," I wrote that day, "knowing that a person had to lose his or her life for me to have this journey. I thank that person and the family for understanding the importance of organ donation, and I will be forever in their debt. God's blessings be with them, and may they find strength, peace, and comfort in knowing that many lives were saved because of their generosity."

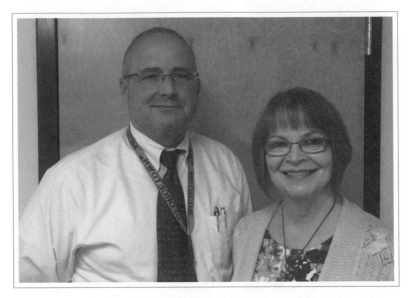

Jill reunites with her transplant surgeon, Dr. Douglas Hale.
Photo by Fred Sauceman.

"Cold night in Nashville," Fred wrote in his reporter's note-book. "Perfect night for Hattie B's Hot Chicken, with pimento cheese macaroni and cheese and collards on the side." Fred brought me back the same sides, boosting my calcium and magnesium! The next night, Saturday night, I did indeed order a big cheese pizza and a Coca-Cola.

14

EATING SALT AND GIVING THANKS

—— JILL ——

After a quiet weekend in the hotel, we returned to Vanderbilt on Monday for my first follow-up appointment with my nephrologist, Dr. Concepcion, and representatives from the Vanderbilt Pharmacy.

"The great thing about you is, number one, you were never on dialysis, and you went straight ahead with what we call a preemptive transplant, and that's really the situation where we see the best outcomes," Dr. Concepcion told me. "And then you got what we call a zero antigen mismatch kidney, which is, despite the antibodies that you have, the best we could hope for as well. What really keeps me in this field is being able to make a difference in someone's life and being a part of this journey, such as yours, and knowing my work has a positive impact. It's patients like you who make me really happy to be doing what I'm doing."

Dr. Concepcion told me that there are more than 100,000 people on the waiting list for kidneys in the United States, and only about 17,000 kidney transplants are performed each year. Around 11,000 of those are from deceased donors. "Only one-tenth of people who need transplants get a deceased donor kidney, and they do often end up waiting five years or more," she added. As Thanksgiving approached that year, I constantly counted my blessings.

Throughout my hospitalization at Vanderbilt and beyond, I was deeply impressed by the fact that members of my healthcare team talked with each other. They always made me feel like I was the only patient they were seeing that day. It may sound like

a simple thing, but sometimes in the health-care arena, that kind
of communication doesn't happen. In my case, pharmacists talked
to nephrologists who talked to surgeons who talked to nurses, as
information was shared openly at every stage. My return visits
always begin with blood work and a urine sample early in the
morning. By the time of my appointment at 10:00 A.M., most of
those test results are available and the doctor reviews them with
me in the office. Testing Prograf levels takes a little longer, but typically by the time we get to Knoxville on our way home, that information is posted on my patient portal and I can view it online. "I'm
on my computer all the time unless I'm doing rounds or seeing
patients," Dr. Concepcion told me.

Another article appeared in the *Johnson City Press* the weekend
before I came home. The online version included a photograph
of nurse Yerus Abebe and me, taken the day after surgery. I was
thrilled to see her get such recognition. I didn't have time to apply
makeup for the photo, but in this case, that was okay. While we
were in the hotel, WCYB-TV reporter Olivia Caridi called to set
up another interview, which we did in our home back in Johnson
City on Wednesday. She shot video of me cooking breakfast and
interviewed me about my transplant experience.

On our November 25 visit back to Vanderbilt, thirty-four
staples were taken out of my ten-inch-long incision. In the hallway
of the Vanderbilt clinic that day, we ran into Julius Blevins and his
wife, Diana, the Saltville, Virginia, couple we had met that very
first day back in August of 2013. They shared the great news that
Julius would be getting a kidney from his cousin the next month,
one week before Christmas.

Thanksgiving that year was on November 27. In years past, we
had hosted huge dinners at our house, sometimes with as many
as forty people. In 2014, it was just Fred and me, as he cooked a
panful of turkey piccata. But with the constant emails, calls, and
Facebook well wishes we were getting, it felt like our home was
filled with people for that most special of Thanksgiving holidays.
The doorbell rang once that day, and it was Glen Whittington, our

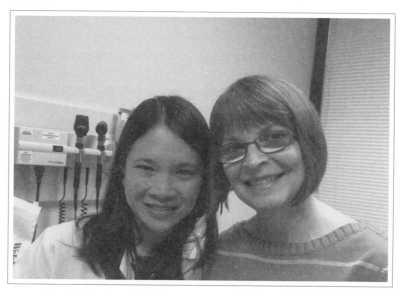

Vanderbilt nephrologist Dr. Beatrice Concepcion with Jill at her
first post-hospital checkup. Photo by Fred Sauceman.

contractor, and his wife, Dot, bearing pumpkin pie and homemade
ice cream, on the day before they were to celebrate sixty years of
marriage.

I made a note after my December 1 checkup at Vanderbilt: "Eat
salt." This chronic sufferer from hypertension was now having to
increase sodium intake to raise my blood pressure! Four weeks
after surgery, I retired the "urine hat," no longer having to measure
input and output. Taking my temperature and weighing myself
every day weren't required anymore, and checking my blood pressure was only necessary twice a day. I was off all medications to
control it.

On December 9, my creatinine had fallen to 0.87, the lowest
since my surgery. That day, I underwent a minor procedure in the
office of urologist Dr. Daniel Barocas to remove the tube that had
connected the ureter to the bladder. This small tube helped to keep
the flow of urine into the bladder until the ureter had time to heal.

My visits to Vanderbilt included time with dietitian Jane Greene, who coached me to eat more dark green vegetables, whole grains, nuts, and dairy products to improve my magnesium and phosphorus levels. "No matter how hard you try to eat foods high in magnesium, your antirejection medicines and Nexium are going to pull it out of you," said the personable Jane, adding that she wasn't "the food police." I bought pumpkin seeds by the pound and followed her prescribed regimen.

"It's challenging to think of creative ways to help people find the right food to eat, to help people understand the role they have in preserving their kidney function or taking care of their transplant," Jane told us. "I admire your ability to do what you did with your diet before your transplant with absolutely no help. Some people have the initiative, but so many people don't. You were proactive and jumped in and did it yourself. We're lucky you didn't restrict protein too much and you weren't so malnourished. What you did is a reflection of the academic background in your house—the curiosity about food and recipes that you all have. I'm not surprised you did it. You have the interest and ability to do research. The first time that I saw you after transplant and you told me what all you did on your own, I was very impressed. That makes you unique.

"Changing eating habits is very, very hard," Jane continued. "Food is involved in everything—day-to-day activities, family meals, celebrations, holidays. That's the way it is until we die. And when we die, we're there in the coffin and everybody else is eating the food that's brought in by all the people to comfort you. It never stops."

By December 23, after I followed Jane's advice, my magnesium level was just above normal. Phosphorus and potassium were right in the middle of the normal range.

I felt well enough to return to the kitchen, where I made crockpot candy for my doctors and nurses at Vanderbilt.

CROCKPOT CANDY

4 ounces of German baking chocolate broken into squares

12 ounces of semisweet baking chocolate broken into squares

24 ounces of white almond bark coating broken into squares

A 16-ounce jar of roasted salted peanuts

A 16-ounce jar of roasted unsalted or lightly salted peanuts

Put chocolate and white bark coating in a crockpot in the order listed. Add peanuts. Cook on low for three hours. Do not do anything to the mixture for the three hours. Then stir thoroughly until well-blended. Drop onto waxed paper using a soup spoon. When the candy has hardened, store it in an airtight container.

"One more thing," I wrote on December 23. "The nurse practitioner [April DeMers] said my antibody levels have not changed since before I had the transplant, which means there is no sign of my body trying to reject this kidney. It is the best Christmas present ever."

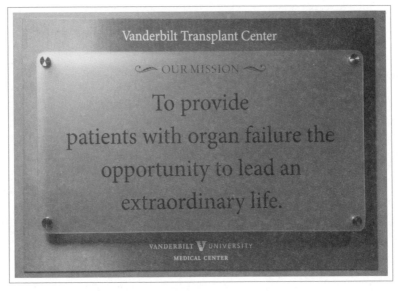

Mission accomplished. Photo by Fred Sauceman.

AFTERWORD:
THE CASE FOR ORGAN DONATION

- 117,000 people were on the national transplant waiting list as of July 2017.

- 33,611 transplants were performed in 2016.

- 22 people die each day waiting for a transplant.

- Nearly six in ten donors are deceased and four in ten are living donors.

WHY IT'S IMPORTANT TO REGISTER TO BE AN ORGAN DONOR

- 95 percent of US adults support organ donation, but only 54 percent are actually signed up as donors.

- Every ten minutes another person is added to the waiting list.

- Only three in 1,000 people die in a way that allows for organ donation.

- One person can donate up to eight lifesaving organs.

- 82.9 percent of prospective transplant recipients are waiting on a kidney.

12.3 percent are waiting on a liver.

3.4 percent are waiting on a heart.

1.2 percent are waiting on a lung.

2.5 percent are all other organs.

(Note: The total is more than 100 percent due to patients included in multiple categories. Organ donation statistics from organdonor.gov US Government information on organ donation and transplantation.)

—— DR. DOUGLAS HALE ——
Transplant Surgeon

There's a massive need for organs. The problem is, how do you convince people to overcome personal biases, cultural biases, and how do you convince them to do that at a time of immense grief, to agree to organ donation? This is the problem that the country has been dealing with for the last twenty years. Still, a lot of organs wind up getting buried that could have been used. How do you fix that? You make people more aware of the need. I think you really work hard to make sure that the system for allocating organs is transparent and fair because the minute people think that something is rigged in somebody else's favor, then they're going to lose interest in donating. You have to publicize the success stories to show people what a difference it does make. It's a lot easier, I think, to take a small child with a liver or heart transplant and to show the transformation in them and the future that they have, but the same benefit is conferred to everyone no matter what they get—either a cornea, kidney, or pancreas. It is a life-transforming event. We must make sure people understand that these organs are equitably distributed. Until the time comes when we can grow them, either in a barnyard or in a test tube, this is going to be the limiting factor.

—— APRIL DEMERS ——
Nurse Practitioner

I think what I would say to most people is, one, it's a personal decision, and any decision that's made for organ donation needs to be made without coercion and without guilt. And you need to always have the freedom to change your mind at any point if you decide it's not for you. The nice thing about kidneys is you have two. Everyone is perfectly capable of functioning with one. And if it's well taken care of, it will last most people the rest of their lives, so you're not taking away the capability of the person who donates to live a full life. Part of the pitch is it's major surgery, so it has potential for complication and decreased quality of life for certain periods of time. When you donate, especially from a deceased donor, sometimes the only solace people have in tragedies is to know that other people were given a second chance. It sometimes is the only thing that brings comfort. Ultimately it's giving someone a second chance at life who has no other options, except for dialysis, and even dialysis long-term is dangerous. You get to take people that otherwise may not live a week, six months, a year—you basically have a death sentence when you have end organ failure. What transplant allows us to do is to take those people and give them a new life.

EPILOGUE

— JILL —

My kidney function is holding its own with the creatinine reading between 0.9 and 1.0. If I never did before, I now truly believe in miracles. The unfortunate event in this miracle is that someone's son, brother, father, grandson, or uncle had to lose his life in the process. I have written a letter to the donor family expressing my condolences and thanking them for their generous gift. It was the hardest letter I have ever written because my joy is possible only through a family's sadness. I hope that they find comfort in knowing their loved one lives on through me.

Amid the joy and celebration, there are some very important requirements for all transplant patients. Because of the antirejection medications I take, I am more susceptible to cancer, in particular skin cancer. Therefore, I see my dermatologist, Dr. Robert Clemons, several times a year, wear protective clothing, and use sun block. I keep up-to-date on my yearly mammogram and pelvic exams and have a colonoscopy every five years. Another requirement for transplant patients is to have a bone density screening every two years.

Over time, a transplant patient's antirejection medication may be reduced, depending on how well the patient is doing and the levels in the blood. When I first began taking Prograf (one of the antirejection medications) after the transplant, my dosage was 6 milligrams every 12 hours. I am now down to 1.5 milligrams every 12 hours, which maintains the proper levels in my blood. I will also have to take 5 milligrams of prednisone for the life of the kidney. Except for some medication adjustments to thwart side effects in the beginning, I have never had any problems with medications.

Vaccinations are very important for transplant patients, and every year I get my flu vaccine. I had a pneumonia vaccine a few months after the transplant surgery and will receive another at age 65. Transplant patients cannot have vaccines made with a live virus, such as the shingles vaccine. With a suppressed immune system from the antirejection drugs, the risk of potentially getting sick from that virus would be too great.

I cannot stress enough the importance of drinking plenty of water every day. As a young child and teenager, I did not do that, and it was probably another reason that lupus settled in my kidneys. All I ever wanted to drink while growing up was milk and Pepsi-Cola. In high school, I switched to iced tea. When I was sick with pneumonia and sinus infections, my mother said that was all she could get me to drink. I drank iced tea until my thirties, when I had trouble with a rapid heart rate. My doctor recommended coming off all caffeine. At that point, I finally turned to water. During the ten years prior to my transplant, I was known all around the community as "the water lady." I carried a huge jug of water with me everywhere, even to church. With my failing kidneys, I did not have problems getting rid of fluid. The effect that lupus had on my kidneys was in filtering waste products, which built up in my body instead of being carried out through the urine. So I drank plenty of water, hoping it would help keep my kidneys flushed out and functioning. But it was too little, too late. Had I been properly hydrated when I was young, the outcome may have been different. I will not make that mistake again. As the medical staff at Vanderbilt instructed, I drink two to three liters of water every day.

Now, for the first time in a long time, I feel like I can lead a fairly normal life. My husband and I love to experience food from other cultures as well as the food of our native Appalachia and the South. Among our many activities, we write food articles for *Blue*

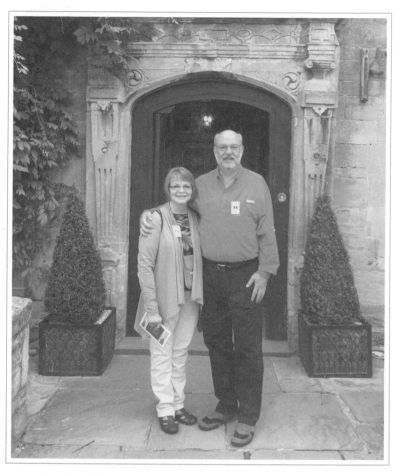

Our first trip to England, at the Lygon Arms Hotel in Broadway.

Ridge Country magazine, and Fred writes for *Smoky Mountain Living* as well. We travel around the region often to do research for those articles and for the books Fred writes. I am so fortunate to have the energy and appetite to participate fully in this work. However, I do have to watch fat and sugar content and pace myself when eating meals. People often ask us why we don't weigh 300 pounds. My answer is that I don't eat everything on my plate. I sample, bringing leftovers home for another meal.

Travel has always been one of our beloved pastimes, and now that I feel like it, I am taking advantage of every opportunity. In fact, I took my first trip abroad in the summer of 2016, traveling around England. I felt comfortable eating the food there without any fear of food-borne illnesses. Vomiting and diarrhea are the greatest risks to kidney transplant patients, due to the loss of fluids. Fortunately, I haven't experienced them. But I have been told that if either should occur, to go to the ER so IV fluids can be administered.

In May of 2017, we became the parents of two miniature schnauzer puppies, Fritz and Sofie. Dogs were always a part of my husband's life and were a part of most of our married life. When we lost our 18-year-old Yorkiepoo, Lucy, we knew eventually we would have another pet when the right time came around. It has been a joy to watch Fritz and Sofie grow and learn. Puppies are just like babies, up at all hours of the night. There is no way I would have had the energy to care for them prior to the kidney transplant.

Down the road, I will need my forty-year-old hip prostheses revised since they are both loose. I see an orthopedist, Vanderbilt's Dr. Andrew Shinar, on a yearly basis for an assessment. So far, they don't cause much pain, and as long as I'm not having lots of problems, the doctor and I have agreed to wait. When I do have the revision surgery, I want to have it done at Vanderbilt in case of any complications.

Adjusting daily living practices, adhering to medication schedules, and keeping all doctors' appointments are lifetime requirements for transplant patients. But it's such a small price to pay in order to have a second opportunity to live life to the fullest. Yes, there are risks to taking those medications. But I choose not to think about those risks, move forward, do everything I can to avoid the risks, and then deal with them should they arise.

It has been forty-four years since I first heard the term "lupus." During these years I have had three major lupus flares and probably lots of little ones. Unfortunately, the last one did the irreversible damage to my kidneys. But I am happy to say that I have not been caught by the "wolf" since 2004. Once a woman goes through menopause, it very seldom rears its ugly head again. But it can happen. It is even more important now, with my new kidney, to keep a close watch for a possible lupus flare. Even though medications I take keep lupus in remission, they are not a cure. The situation is the same with a kidney transplant. It is a treatment for kidney failure, not a cure. I see my rheumatologist, Dr. Lurie, every six months for blood work and checkups. So even if this "wolf" starts chasing me again, I believe I can outrun him.

Throughout this life with lupus nephritis, I have tried to keep a positive attitude and have faith that God will see me through each situation. I remember an appointment with my primary care physician when he was reviewing my medical history with an intern. The intern was amazed at how well I seemed to look after hearing all about the lupus and kidney disease. My doctor said that he had patients with far less wrong with them than me and they were in worse shape. He looked at the intern and said, "I truly believe it's because of Jill's positive attitude. She chooses to see the cup half full instead of half empty, and she feels fortunate for what she is able to do. She knows that God will help her deal with whatever she has been handed." And so He has!

Appendix A

WHAT IS CHRONIC KIDNEY DISEASE?

Chronic kidney disease (CKD) is a condition characterized by a gradual loss of kidney function over time. If kidney disease gets worse, wastes can build to high levels in your blood and make you feel sick. Also, kidney disease increases your risk of having heart and blood vessel disease.

Thirty million American adults have CKD and millions of others are at increased risk. Early detection can help prevent the progression of kidney disease to kidney failure. The two main causes of CKD are diabetes and high blood pressure, which are responsible for two-thirds of the cases. Other conditions that affect the kidneys are glomerulonephritis, inherited diseases such as polycystic kidney disease, malformations of the kidney, lupus and other autoimmune diseases, obstructions such as kidney stones or tumors, and repeated urinary infections. Two simple tests can detect CKD: urine albumin and serum creatinine.

Severe symptoms may not develop until the advanced stages of CKD. However, you may notice that you:

- Feel more tired and have less energy
- Have trouble concentrating
- Have a poor appetite
- Have trouble sleeping
- Have muscle cramping at night
- Have swollen feet and ankles
- Have puffiness around your eyes, especially in the morning
- Have dry, itchy skin
- Need to urinate more often, especially at night

Source: The National Kidney Foundation

Appendix B

THE FIVE STAGES OF KIDNEY FAILURE

Stage 1: Normal or high GFR greater than 90 mL/min. No symptoms. Found when being tested for another condition. Treatment: eat a healthy diet, keep blood pressure at healthy level, keep blood sugar or diabetes under control, have regular checkups that include a serum creatinine to measure GFR, take medicines as prescribed, exercise regularly, and stop smoking.

Stage 2: Mild kidney damage with a GFR of 60–89 mL/min. No symptoms. Found when being tested for another condition. Same treatment options as for stage 1.

Stage 3A: Moderately reduced kidney function with a GFR of 45–59 mL/min.

Stage 3B: Moderately reduced kidney function with a GFR of 30–44 mL/min. Symptoms include fatigue, fluid retention and swelling, shortness of breath, urine changes (foamy, dark orange, brown, tea-colored, or red), urinating more or less than normal, kidney pain felt in the back, and sleep problems.

Patient should see a nephrologist to offer the best advice for treatment to help keep kidneys working as long as possible. Diet changes will consist of limiting foods that contain phosphorus, especially processed foods with phosphorus additives; eating high quality protein foods; possibly limiting potassium; consuming whole grains, fruits, and vegetables; balancing carbohydrates; decreasing saturated fats; lowering sodium; and limiting calcium. Medications should be taken exactly as prescribed. Exercise regularly and stop smoking.

Stage 4: Advanced kidney damage with a severe decrease in GFR to 15–30 mL/min. It is likely someone in this stage will eventually need dialysis or a kidney transplant in the near future. Because of waste products building up in the blood, this person is likely to develop complications such as high blood pressure, anemia, bone disease, heart disease, and other cardiovascular diseases.

Symptoms: All those of stage 3 plus nausea and/or vomiting, taste changes such as a metallic taste in the mouth, bad breath, loss of appetite, difficulty concentrating, and nerve problems.

It is necessary to see a nephrologist at least every three months for blood tests. The nephrologist will also discuss the forms of dialysis as well as talk about kidney transplantation. This patient will be referred to a dietitian to recommend a meal plan individualized for his or her needs and one that usually includes reducing protein intake. It is very important to take blood pressure, diabetes, and other medications as prescribed by your doctor. Exercise regularly and do not smoke.

Stage 5: Called end-stage renal disease (ESRD). The GFR is 15 mL/min or below. The kidneys have lost nearly all their ability to do their job effectively, and eventually dialysis or a transplant is needed to live.

Symptoms include loss of appetite, nausea or vomiting, headaches, fatigue, inability to concentrate, itching, making little or no urine, swelling around eyes and ankles, muscle cramps, tingling in hands or feet, changes in skin color, and increased skin pigmentation.

The kidneys are no longer able to regulate blood pressure, produce the hormone that helps make red blood cells, or activate vitamin D for healthy bones. Your nephrologist will develop your overall care plan to manage your health-care team. You will be referred to a dialysis center and, if you wish, to a transplant center to be evaluated for the kidney transplant waiting list.

Source: DaVita Kidney Care

Appendix C

WHY DO SOME PEOPLE WAIT LONGER THAN OTHERS FOR A TRANSPLANT?

Waiting time for a kidney can depend on factors such as:

ABO (blood type). Blood type O has the longest wait. This is because blood type O donors can donate to other blood groups, but a patient with blood type O can only receive an organ from a donor with blood type O. Also, it has been found that those with blood type B tend to have longer wait times as well.

Prior pregnancies, blood transfusions, or past transplants. Those increase a substance in your body called antibodies. A higher level of antibodies in your blood can make it more difficult to match with a compatible donor.

Changes to the US organ allocation system in December 2014 have had an impact on the way kidneys are allocated to patients. These changes to the wait-list have allowed some flexibility with the factors listed above. For example, donor matching is now done to more closely match the age of the donor and recipient. This means a kidney coming from a 30-year-old donor will more likely go to someone in that age range. This is called longevity matching.

Another big change that was made has to do with patients who joined the wait-list after being on dialysis. You now build wait-time from the time that you started dialysis—or when it is documented that your GFR dropped to below 20—instead of the date when you were placed on the waiting list.

Finally, extra priority is now given to patients who are extraordinarily hard to match because of having high levels of antibodies from prior transplants, blood transfusions, or pregnancies.

Source: The National Kidney Foundation

Appendix D

USEFUL RESOURCES

Alliance for Paired Donation
www.paireddonation.org

Donate Life America and the National Donate Life Registry
www.donatelife.net
www.registerme.org

Lupus Foundation of America
www.lupus.org

National Kidney Foundation
www.kidney.org

National Kidney Foundation Living Donors Program
www.livingdonors.org

United Network for Organ Sharing
www.unos.org

Vanderbilt Transplant Center
www.vanderbilttransplantcenter.com

Appendix E

FINANCIAL ASSISTANCE FOR LIVING DONORS AND TRANSPLANT RECIPIENTS

Air Care Alliance

www.aircareall.org

May be able to provide free or low-cost flights for medical evaluation and surgery for living donors and recipients.

American Kidney Fund

www.akfinc.org

Provides limited grants to needy dialysis patients, kidney transplant recipients, and living kidney donors to help cover the costs of health-related expenses, transportation, and medication.

National Living Donor Assistance Center

www.livingdonorassistance.org

May be able to pay up to a certain amount for the living donor's (and his or her companions') travel and lodging expenses.

Donors and recipients should also ask their transplant centers about assistance with financial issues.

ACKNOWLEDGMENTS

Hundreds of skilled hands and caring hearts have made this story possible. We thank our parents, Elsie Derting and the late Homer Derting and the late Fred and Wanda Sauceman, who created loving homes for us and rich childhood memories and experiences that continue to shape us and guide us today. We thank Jill's sisters, Joyce and Janice, who often had to take a backseat as Jill's medical care took priority in the family. Along with Jill's parents, Joyce spent many hours sitting with her in hospital rooms.

We say thank you multiplied many times over to someone whose identity, at the time of this writing, we don't even know— the 27-year-old man who gave the kidney to save Jill's life. We thank another hero we do know, Myles Cook, who stepped up to donate a kidney and who had gotten so far into the process that fall of 2014 that we consider him a "donor," too. He provided hope at a time when it had begun to wane for us.

Dr. Jerry Miller, then in Nickelsville, Virginia, made that initial diagnosis of lupus in 1974, at a time when the disease was still somewhat of a mystery. We also thank the doctors at Associated Orthopedics in Kingsport for their knowledge and skill in performing total hip replacements: the late Dr. Joseph Maloy, Dr. Robert T. Strang Sr., and Dr. Robert T. Strang Jr.

Nephrologist Dr. Clifford Wiegand in Johnson City is not only a fine physician but also a keen listener. His wisdom in listening to the patient is largely responsible for Jill having been able to avoid dialysis. Dr. David Lurie is without doubt one of the finest rheumatologists in the country, and we are so fortunate that he has chosen to practice in our community, Johnson City, Tennessee. Dr.

Jason Hatjioannou is another hometown treasure, who now serves as Jill's primary care physician.

We will be eternally grateful to Jill's transplant surgeon, Dr. Douglas Hale at Vanderbilt, for her highly successful outcome, and we appreciate and admire the talent and knowledge of nephrologist Dr. Beatrice Concepcion at Vanderbilt, who continues to help us nurture this kidney. She has become a great friend, too. Usually her very first question during an appointment is, "Where did you eat last night?"

So many people at Vanderbilt University Medical Center and its Renal Transplant Clinic contributed to the success of Jill's transplant. It is a joy to visit them, and we look forward to every appointment. In particular, we thank transplant nurses Yerus Abebe, April DeMers, Kristin Smith, and Ashley Wilson. From Vanderbilt's 7th floor Critical Care Unit, we thank Jessica Walker and a nurse we know only as Elizabeth.

Dr. J. Kelly Smith, now retired from the Department of Internal Medicine at East Tennessee State University's Quillen College of Medicine, took over Jill's case at a critical time and guided her through the pain of a major lupus flare. We appreciate all his many kindnesses.

Dr. Paul E. Stanton Jr., President Emeritus of East Tennessee State University and a member of the Tennessee Health Care Hall of Fame, has been a valued friend and confidante since the 1980s. From the day of Jill's transplant and for about two weeks after, he called to check on her every day.

We thank the following doctors who have also followed Jill's case over the years: Drs. David Goldman, Ronald Irby, Barbara Kimbrough, Steven Lloyd, Marsha Sentell, and Ron Sinicrope. We thank the staff at the Johnson City Medical Center and Holston Valley Community Hospital in Kingsport. We appreciate our insurance company, Blue Cross Blue Shield of Tennessee, for its efficiency and professionalism.

We are grateful to our church families, past and present— Weber City Christian Church in Virginia, Asbury United

Methodist Church in Greeneville, and to the churches in Scott County, Virginia, whose congregations assisted Jill and her family spiritually and financially in the 1970s. Our current church, Jonesborough Presbyterian, has been a source of great inspiration and support. We thank every member of that congregation, led by former pastor Dr. Beth Yarborough, interim pastor Dr. Conrad Crow, and current pastor Allen Huff. Cherry Smith, the church's brilliant music director, and the Jonesborough Presbyterian church choir have played a special role in Jill's return to singing.

We thank Tina Graham for her steadfast friendship and for taking the lead in creating the Facebook page "Jill's Journey: Quest for a Kidney," which we have renamed "Jill's Journey: Successful Quest for a Kidney."

Our gratitude goes out to our colleagues at ETSU and WETS-FM for standing with us through these experiences. We are indebted to the members of the news media in East Tennessee and Southwest Virginia for their friendship and for helping us let the people of our region know that Jill was in dire need of a kidney. Thanks to longtime ETSU photographer Larry Smith for his assistance with pictures.

Jennifer Wetzel and her colleagues in the Vanderbilt University Office of News and Communications kindly arranged our interviews with the medical professionals at Vanderbilt who contributed greatly to the content of this book.

Aunts, uncles, cousins, friends, and coworkers all played a part in this story. Through Facebook, friends have followed and encouraged us from all over the world. We thank Brenda Murray, who has worked for us for more than thirty years and who took care of our home during the many trips to Nashville and through countless other hospital visits. We thank Glen Whittington for all the improvements he made in our home and his wife, Dot, for her friendship, too, as well as her hot rolls. We thank our "honorary grandmother," the late Marguerite Keefauver, dorm mother at Carter Hall, for approving of Fred and for taking part in our wedding in 1980.

Our frequent trips to Nashville have allowed us to reconnect with friends Jimmy and Denise Mitchell, who showed up in our various hotel rooms bearing gift bags full of kidney-healthy snacks and who have joined us in reacquainting ourselves with the food of Nashville, from hot chicken to Turkish eggplant salad.

For allowing us to share this story in book form, we are deeply grateful to the talented staff at Mercer University Press in Macon, Georgia: Marc Jolley, Marsha Luttrell, Mary Beth Kosowski, Jenny Toole, and Heather Comer. On behalf of anyone who might find comfort, encouragement, and hope through our story, we thank you.

Jill and Fred Sauceman
Johnson City, Tennessee
July 2017